'The Sirtfood Diet shows the amazing benefits of plant-based foods and celebrates them at their best with easy and satisfying recipes for vegetarians and vegans.'

Mary McCartney, photographer

'The change has been amazing. I feel much more active, energetic – it doesn't feel like a diet because I have changed my eating habits for life.'

Laurenne, in remission from breast cancer, lost 20lb (9kg) in six weeks

'Thank you! My husband is looking extra hot.'

The wife of one of the Sirtfood Diet participants after he lost 7lb 8oz (3.4kg) in 7 days

'The initial day was tough, but after that I felt my energy levels surge and I slept better. I think one challenging day is worth a lifetime of health.'

James M., lost 7lb 4oz (3.3kg) in 7 days

'The diet got me in the shape of my life just in time for my wedding day.'

Jadis T., lost over 6lb (2.7kg) including gaining 2lb (900g) of muscle in 7 days

'It might just be a lifesaver.'

David C., lost over 24lb (11kg) and reversed metabolic disease in 6 months

Aidan Goggins

Driven by his quest to cure his own rare autoimmune disease, Aidan is, unusually, both a pharmacist and nutritionist. It is this unique mix that has led to Aidan becoming one of Europe's most sought-after health experts, with clients ranging from doctors to celebrity personalities. A huge fitness enthusiast, he specialises in sports nutrition, and his dietary expertise underpins the success of many champion professional athletes. Aidan is a prominent health commentator in the media as well as an award-winning writer.

Glen Matten

With a master's degree in nutritional medicine and a passion for good food, Glen is an accomplished author whose books include the award-winning *The Health Delusion* and bestselling *The Sirtfood Diet*. Glen makes frequent forays into the media, spanning TV, radio and numerous national magazines and newspapers. With an approach deeply rooted in nutritional science, Glen has run successful clinics across the UK for over a decade. He collaborates closely with medical doctors, attracts clients from all over the world, and works with a number of professional athletes and celebrities.

Mark McCulloch

Mark McCulloch has been a professional chef for 25 years. He is passionate about creating healthy food without compromising on flavour, and helped to create the recipes for the original Sirtfood diet.

the sirt food diet

RECIPE BOOK

AIDAN GOGGINS & GLEN MATTEN
With Chef MARK McCULLOCH

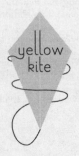

yellow kite

First published in Great Britain in 2016 by Yellow Kite
An imprint of Hodder & Stoughton
An Hachette UK company

1

A CIP catalogue record for this title is available from the British Library.

Trade Paperback ISBN 978 1 473 63858 7
Ebook ISBN 978 1 473 63857 0

Typeset in Sabon MT by Palimpsest Book Production Limited,
Falkirk, Stirlingshire
Printed and bound by CPI Group UK Ltd, Croydon, CR0 4YY

The advice here is not intended to replace the services of trained health professionals
or to be a substitute for medical advice. You are advised to consult with your
healthcare professional with regards to matters relating to your health, and in
particular regarding matters that may require diagnosis or medical attention.

Hodder & Stoughton policy is to use papers that are natural,
renewable and recyclable products and made from wood grown in
sustainable forests. The logging and manufacturing processes are expected
to conform to the environmental regulations of the country of origin.

Hodder & Stoughton Ltd
Carmelite House
50 Victoria Embankment
London EC4Y 0DZ

www.hodder.co.uk

Contents

Introduction

When we first started investigating the idea that the naturally occurring chemicals found in plants could be the answer to our modern-day health woes, we had no idea we were stumbling across what could quite possibly be the biggest nutrition breakthrough for health and weight loss of modern times. In fact, having received critical acclaim as two serious nutritionists who debunked weight-loss diets, we were just about the last people who would ignite a best-selling diet phenomenon that would cause ingredient shortages in supermarkets across the country.

Looking back on the runaway success of *The Sirtfood Diet*, we think it's actually because we are such diet sceptics that readers have embraced our ideas all the more enthusiastically. After all, we'd be the first to tell you that it's well proven that 99 per cent of dieters fail to lose weight in the long term, with most of them ending up heavier than they started. As much as people want to believe in diets, deep down we know they simply offer empty promises.

With *The Sirtfood Diet*, we've done something very different. As busy clinicians with a combined 25 years' experience treating patients, one thing has always struck us. In our experience, a healthy weight and long-term well-being are achieved only by consuming the foods and nutrients our bodies need, not through deprivation. If we can provide these much-needed nutrients through delicious foods and recipes that bring joy and pleasure back to mealtimes, then we are truly on to something great that will change for good the way we approach the food we eat. And that is the essence of what this book is all about.

Changing the way we think

Anything that changes the landscape of how we think and approach diet will inevitably meet early resistance. We saw it with our first book, *The Health Delusion*, a scathing critique of the flaws of the diet and supplement industry, and our take on what really works. Initially slammed by those with vested interests or rigidly stuck in their ways, these critics were quickly silenced as every relevant large nutrition study that was published subsequently supported the case we made. In the end, with the evidence overwhelming, the book won industry and critical acclaim, along with a health book of the year award, and some of those early vocal critics are now among our strongest allies. *The Sirtfood Diet* is no different. We are making the bold claim that yes we should be encouraged to eat more plant foods, but if we want to specifically promote weight loss with optimal well-being, then it's time to realise that not all plant foods (including fruit and vegetables) are equal.

This is a radical idea that runs counter to the prevailing dogma of our times. It is no longer good enough to cling to the generic advice that tells us just to eat five portions of fruit and vegetables a day as part of a balanced diet. We need only look around us to see how little impact that has had. In fact, we now know when it comes to health, many foods that the supposed health experts warned us away from, such as chocolate, coffee and tea, trump most fruits and vegetables out there. *The Sirtfood Diet* has revolutionised the standard recommendations for fruit and vegetables and forced us to look far beyond their content of vitamins, minerals and antioxidants. Instead, we present the provocative idea that the benefits of plant foods are mostly down to their sirtuin-activating nutrient content.

Such a fundamental challenge to the way we think will undoubtedly ruffle the feathers of those with a vested interest in maintaining the status quo. So we were delighted to see that within one month of the release of *The Sirtfood*

Diet a paper* in the prestigious *British Medical Journal* reported on research carried out at Harvard University that gave strong support to these claims. Researchers analysed the dietary habits and plant consumption of just over 124,000 Americans over 24 years. They found that it was only certain plants, those rich in natural plant chemicals called polyphenols, that promoted healthy weight. Other fruits and vegetables that lacked appreciable amounts of these specific polyphenols had no beneficial effect on weight. It will likely come as no surprise that the plant chemicals found to have benefit for weight are those found in Sirtfoods. Welcome to the revolution.

Putting the Sirt into food

We've known for years that eating more plant foods reduces disease, even if we didn't fully understand why. With our own backgrounds in nutritional medicine and pharmacy, we were also very aware that the powerful constituents of certain plants form the basis of many of today's most effective drugs for treating major diseases such as heart disease, diabetes and even cancer. We knew plants were powerful stuff. But it was in 2013 that we really stood up

* Bertoia, M.L. et al, 'Dietary flavonoid intake and weight maintenance: three prospective cohorts of 124 086 US men and women followed for up to 24 years', *BMJ* 352:i17 (2016)

and started asking big questions. This was when a game-changing study of the Mediterranean diet, called Predimed, was published. It was conducted on almost 7,400 individuals at high risk of cardiovascular disease, and the results were so good that the trial was actually stopped early – after just five years. The premise of Predimed was beautifully simple. It asked what would be the difference between a Mediterranean-style diet supplemented with either extra virgin olive oil or nuts (especially walnuts) compared to a more conventional modern-day diet? And what a difference it was. The change in diet reduced the incidence of cardiovascular disease by around 30 per cent, a result drug companies can only dream of. Upon further follow-up it was found that there was also a 30 per cent fall in diabetes, along with significant drops in inflammation, improvements in memory and brain health, as well as a 40 per cent reduction in the likelihood of becoming obese.

Yet researchers were unable to explain clearly what produced these dramatic benefits. Neither the amount of calories, fats nor sugars eaten – the typical measures used to grade the food we eat – differed enough between the groups to affect the outcome. There was something else going on.

Then the eureka moment struck. Separately, a whole new area of exciting research was being undertaken in the world of sirtuin genes. Our sirtuin genes, also called our 'skinny genes', are a group of special genes in the body which, when turned on, activate a recycling process in our cells that clears

5

out the cellular debris and clutter that accumulates over time and causes ill health and loss of vitality. To fuel this recycling process the body uses our fat cells. The result is that when we activate our sirtuin genes, not only do we increase our sense of well-being, we also increase our resistance to disease and burn significant amounts of fat in the process. Think of it as triggering the holy trinity of health.

For years we have known that there are two ways to activate our sirtuin genes: fasting and exercise, yet neither is perfect. During fasting we deprive the body of nourishment, which causes it to send out alarm signals that translate into hunger and irritability. We also feel tired and lose muscle due to the lack of fuel. Exercise, while extremely beneficial in moderate amounts, is required in much larger levels to stimulate weight loss. These levels are unsustainable for many, and research now even suggests they are bad for us, making it questionable whether this was the sole way nature intended us to stimulate our sirtuin genes. Then came the discovery of a third way for stimulating our sirtuin genes: food. And with that the landscape of diet and nutrition changed forever.

Bigging up Sirtfoods

Always looking for that multi-billion pound magic bullet drug panacea, the pharmaceutical industry was also investigating our sirtuin genes in the hopes of discovering patentable chemicals that could activate them. Just as they have done for so many new drugs in the past, 'Big Pharma' turned to plants for inspiration. It was in doing so that they discovered something remarkable. They showed that there are naturally occurring nutrients found in plants – a subgroup of what are called polyphenols – that have the tantalising power to turn on our sirtuin genes, just like fasting and exercise. We call the foods with notable quantities of these sirtuin-activating nutrients 'Sirtfoods' and their discovery has become a game changer in how we look to the future of nutrition.

We turned our attention back to the Predimed study and discovered that as part of a Mediterranean diet, both extra virgin olive oil and walnuts stand out for their substantial content of sirtuin-activating nutrients. Essentially, what the researchers had unwittingly created was a Sirtfood-rich diet. Finally we had the explanation to the mind-blowing benefits this study observed. In fact, we soon found this was not unique to just these two foods of the Mediterranean diet. Across the world there are regions dubbed 'Blue Zones', where people not only live longer than in countries where a typical Western diet is the norm, they also remain slim and retain youthful vitality into old age.

Sirtfoods help to explain why this occurs. Whether it is the rich intake of cocoa in the Panama Islands, the copious amounts of green tea and soy consumed in southern Japan, or the liberal use of spices that is synonymous with Indian cuisine, the traditional foods prevalent in these regions are all Sirtfoods.

Since then we have discovered 20 foods with the most significant levels of specific polyphenols that early research has suggested can activate our sirtuin genes. Armed with this knowledge, we asked ourselves: what if we created a special diet that combined all of these foods in exceptionally high quantities? Furthermore, what if we complemented it with moderate fasting to really ramp up sirtuin activation during its initial stages? We tested the diet in 40 individuals at a private gym in London. Stunned by the results, we brought it to the mainstream, and so the Sirtfood Diet was created. The rest, as they say, is history...

Be inspired

Participants in our original trial lost impressive amounts of weight without losing muscle – sometimes actually gaining muscle. Surprisingly, they rarely reported feeling hungry, an outcome we discovered to be unique to the ability of Sirtfoods to regulate appetite. The average weight loss was 7lb (3.2kg) in seven days after accounting for muscle gain. We heard inspiring stories. We heard how people got into perfect shape for their wedding day; we even heard from the wife of a Sirtfood diet participant who contacted us to thank us for transforming her husband, who was now 'looking extra hot'! We were so inspired by the results we were seeing that we started applying these principles to the elite athletes, models and celebrities we worked with regularly, for whom improving body composition and getting lean while feeling fantastic were top priorities. The results we achieved with them were equally stunning.

After *The Sirtfood Diet* was published, more and more inspiring weight-loss success stories poured in. We heard from people who lost up to 11lb (5kg) in the first week and 2 stone (12kg) in the first month. While this in itself was fantastic, as nutritional medicine consultants that specialise in reversing and preventing disease, there was something that inspired us even more: the personal stories that went beyond an improved physique and were nothing short of life-changing. Like the story of Laurenne, who had battled breast cancer but was struggling with the effects of the chemotherapy that caused her weight to balloon and her vitality to hit the floor. Following the Sirtfood Diet helped her to lose 20lb (9kg) in the first six weeks, but best of all it gave her a new lease of life. 'It's been brilliant,' she said. 'The change has been amazing. I feel much more active, energetic – it doesn't feel like a diet because we have changed our eating habits for life.'

Or the story of Robert, who lost 10lb (4.5kg) in just

two weeks but was far more delighted with the dramatic improvements in his mental well-being. In his own words he was now 'loving life'. Since then, there have been many others, from the reversal of menopause symptoms, to improving autoimmune diseases, and even one reader who credited a rapid reversal of the discolouring of the sclera (the white of the eye) to following the Sirtfood Diet.

It's the many stories like these that have inspired us to compile this recipe book to further spread the word that our food choices can be both delicious and life-altering.

Become a Sirtfoodie

We love that you love the selection of recipes we presented in our first *Sirtfood Diet* book. We took even further delight when we saw you applying Sirtfood principles to create your own tasty culinary masterpieces. This is exactly what has spurred us on to develop the much wider selection of recipes that you will find in this book. After all, isn't enjoying the food we eat part and parcel of living life to the full? Who wants austere regimes that constantly restrict us and suck every last drop of pleasure from eating for the rest of their life? Not us, and we don't want that for you either.

The Sirtfood Diet is about *eating* your way to a healthier and leaner body. Our motto is that it's what you put on your plate that matters, not what you take off it. And with that firmly in mind, we want you to join the merry band of Sirtfoodies who revel in eating good food, pack their plates high with Sirtfood delights and don't spend their time fretting about the latest thing they are supposed to be avoiding, or racked with guilt about eating some forbidden pleasure. By adopting the Sirtfood approach, enjoyment of food is never far away. With so many great Sirtfoods at our disposal, an explosion of taste is as good as guaranteed. We don't think there can be too many grounds for complaint with a way of eating that features delicious curry spices, feisty chillies, delectable dark chocolate, sumptuous strawberries and an array of vibrant fresh vegetables and herbs. And did we mention the coffee and red wine?

For those who enjoyed the recipes in *The Sirtfood Diet*, there's now a whole heap more to be enjoyed, which will keep this way of eating fresh and exciting. For those completely new to Sirtfoods, strap in, hold tight and steady yourself for a blitz of big flavours.

What makes up the Sirtfood diet?

PLANTS

Irrespective of whether you are vegetarian or not, plants form the basis of the Sirtfood Diet, and it's worth pausing here to explain why. Every single one of the top 20 Sirtfoods are plant foods and there's a very good reason for that.

Over aeons of evolution, plants have developed a highly sophisticated stress response system to adapt to their environment and survive. They do this by producing a powerful arsenal of natural plant chemicals called polyphenols, which help protect them. When we eat these foods, we also ingest their polyphenols. And we now know that a select group of these natural plant stress chemicals can activate our sirtuin genes. It's the revolutionary idea that we can piggy-back on the stress response of plants for health benefits. It is known as xenohormesis, and is at the heart of the Sirtfood Diet.

The foods with the highest level of these sirtuin-activating polyphenols are called Sirtfoods. We've already mentioned that there are 20 top Sirtfoods and these form the basis of the Sirtfood Diet and feature heavily in the recipes throughout this book. You'll find the complete list on pages 17–20. But we must point out that sirtuin activation is not an all-or-nothing approach. Many other foods have significant amounts of sirtuin-activating nutrients, albeit to a lesser extent than the top 20. Eating a varied and diverse diet is something we strongly encourage, especially as we want you to eat a Sirtfood-rich diet for life. With this in mind, we have also identified an additional 40 foods with meaningful amounts of sirtuin-activating nutrients, which are also incorporated into many of the recipes. These are listed on pages 18–20.

While the pharmaceutical industry is still looking to isolate individual components from plants and synthesise them into a single chemical miracle cure, it's not a vision we share. We know that Sirtfoods are complex foods that work synergistically together. A diet packed full of a combination of Sirtfoods will achieve greater results than any single entity that the pharmaceutical industry can ever patent.

PROTEIN

So, it's plants that put the Sirt into the Sirtfood Diet, but protein is also important, specifically a building block of protein known as leucine, which helps to boost the way Sirtfoods work in the body. This is why, as well as being packed full of Sirtfoods, our recipes also incorporate protein-rich foods.

The good news is that when it comes to where you will get your protein, you can decide. Whether you are a meat fiend, a pescatarian, a plant-only vegan, or, like us, a mixture of all three who love nothing more than to mix and match, we have you covered with ample different options every step of the way.

FATS

The great news is that we've no interest in low-fat anything. We're really not worried about fats, which means you don't need to worry either. In fact, some of our most powerful Sirtfoods, such as extra virgin olive oil and walnuts, are jam-packed with fat, and amazingly good for you. It is their bounty of sirtuin-activating nutrients that matters, not their fat content.

Let the recipes in this book free you from fat phobia once and for all. Some are high in fat, some are low in fat, but that is irrelevant – all are rich in Sirtfoods, which is what counts.

The one type of fat we do keenly encourage in our recipes is omega-3 fish oil. As well as having numerous benefits to health in their own right, these oils also appear to favourably influence the way our sirtuin genes work, making them a very healthful addition.

How this book works

PHASE 1 TO LIFE

The recipes in this book follow the tried-and-trusted formula of our first *Sirtfood Diet* book. That means we kick off with Phase 1, or what we call the 'hyper-success' phase, which is our clinically proven method for losing

7lb (3.2kg) in seven days. But this time there's a vastly expanded repertoire of recipes. You will follow the same step-by-step formula for success, but when it comes to the recipes, there's total flexibility. You get to choose which Phase 1 recipes suit you, your tastes and your lifestyle. Think about it like a recipe pick 'n' mix: meat, fish, vegetarian, quick, slow, gluten-free – you get to choose. What's really great about this more flexible way of doing things is that if you come to repeat Phase 1 for a weight-loss and well-being boost, you can get the same great results but choose a completely different selection of recipes. Or, if you have your trusted favourites, you can just stick with those.

Of course it is not compulsory to do Phase 1. Many of you will already have successfully completed it and are now reaping the benefits of Sirtfood-centric meals as part of your normal eating patterns. This does not mean that you have to miss out on the delicious Phase 1 recipes, however. Think of all the 100 plus recipes in this book as an extension of your current Sirtfood recipe bank for you to embrace the Sirtfood for life experience.

The recipes in the second half of the book are geared towards maintaining and building on the great results achieved in Phase 1. The focus shifts to a balanced way of eating that will not only encourage you to achieve and sustain a healthy weight but bring you lifelong health benefits. Here, the top 20 Sirtfoods still remain centre plate, but we broaden the dietary horizon to include a wider variety of foods that also have Sirtfood properties for a more sustainable way of eating to help keep your body in perfect balance. With recipes for breakfasts, lunches, snacks, dinners and even some desserts thrown in for good measure, it's all about making the Sirtfood way fit into your lifestyle, not vice versa.

TAKE IT EASY OR DO IT IN STYLE

One of the biggest challenges to eating well every day is time, or, to be precise, lack of time. As furiously busy clinicians ourselves, we know just how difficult it can be to stay on top of eating well day in and day out. Add kids, exercise and a social life into the equation and those best-laid plans can quickly evaporate into thin air.

At the same time, we love to cook amazing-tasting food, especially when we have a bit more time to spend in the kitchen or want to make mealtimes with friends or family that bit special. This spurred us on to ensure our recipe range catered to all. Whether you are a culinary neophyte or an emerging cordon bleu chef, we have you covered. And each section of the book contains a good selection of quick and easy options for when time is of the essence. This keeps it do-able for even the busiest of folk. And the one thing we guarantee is that whether it's meals in minutes or recipes that require a bit more TLC, they're all delicious.

WHAT CAN YOU EXPECT?

As well as enjoying some truly delicious food, by following the Sirtfood Diet approach, you can expect to:

- ☑ Lose weight from fat – not muscle
- ☑ Experience long-term weight-loss success
- ☑ Have more energy, look and feel better
- ☑ Feel pleasantly full and satisfied
- ☑ Slash the risk of chronic diseases
- ☑ Live a long and healthy life

So without further ado, it's time to eat your way to the body you've always wanted, one delicious mouthful at a time.

Top 20 Sirtfoods

	Sirtfood	Major sirtuin-activating nutrients
1	Bird's eye chilli	Luteolin, Myricetin
2	Buckwheat	Rutin
3	Capers	Kaempfercl, Quercetin
4	Celery, including its leaves	Apigenin, Luteolin
5	Cocoa	Epicatechin
6	Coffee	Caffeic acid, Chlorogenic acid

7	Extra virgin olive oil	Oleuropein, Hydroxytyrosol
8	Green tea, especially matcha green tea	Epigallocatechin gallate (EGCG)
9	Kale	Kaempferol, Quercetin
10	Lovage	Quercetin
11	Medjool dates	Gallic acid, Caffeic acid
12	Parsley	Apigenin, Myricetin
13	Red chicory	Luteolin
14	Red onion	Quercetin
15	Red wine	Resveratrol, Piceatannol
16	Rocket	Quercetin, Kaempferol
17	Soy	Daidzein, Formononetin
18	Strawberries	Fisetin
19	Turmeric	Curcumin
20	Walnuts	Gallic acid

40 additional foods with Sirtfood properties

Vegetables
- Artichokes
- Asparagus
- Bok choy/pak choi

- Broccoli
- Endive
- Green beans
- Shallots
- Watercress
- White onions
- Yellow chicory

Fruits
- Apples
- Black plums
- Blackberries
- Blackcurrants
- Cranberries
- Goji berries
- Kumquats
- Raspberries
- Red grapes

Nuts and seeds
- Chestnuts
- Chia seeds
- Peanuts
- Pecan nuts
- Pistachio nuts
- Sunflower seeds

Grains and pseudo-grains

- Popping corn
- Quinoa
- Wholemeal flour

Beans

- Broad beans
- White beans (e.g. cannellini or haricot)

Herbs and spices

- Chives
- Dill (fresh and dried)
- Dried oregano
- Dried sage
- Ginger
- Peppermint (fresh and dried)
- Standard chillies/hot peppers
- Thyme (fresh and dried)

Beverages

- Black tea
- White tea

Sirtfood Science: A Recap

We know the more sciency stuff isn't for everyone, so if you're itching to crack on with the Sirtfood Diet plan and recipes, then you can bookmark this chapter for a later date. But if you are like us and love to know a bit about *why* and *how* things work, read on as this is the part of the book where we serve up a healthy slice of Sirtfood science.

One of the things that distinguishes the Sirtfood Diet from just about every diet that has come before is that it focuses on the foods you should be *including* in your diet, not what you should be cutting out. When it comes to nutrition, all we seem to hear nowadays is how much of what we are eating is bad for us. With so much forbidden and so much confusion it's no wonder we find it hard to stick to any of these diets for long. In fact, if you listened to them all, you'd probably want to give up on food altogether.

Now imagine the complete opposite of that: a way of eating that turns all you know on its head, where the benefits for fat-burning and health come from the specific foods you *add* to your diet. These foods are called Sirtfoods.

Sirtuins

To understand how the Sirtfood Diet works we have to touch briefly on genes, specifically, on an ancient family of genes we all have. In fact, you might think of these particular genes as the conductor of some great orchestra, coordinating processes within our cells that influence our ability to burn fat, resist disease and even increase our lifespan. These genes are known as sirtuins and they hold the key to why the Sirtfood Diet is so effective.

What's striking about sirtuins is that they get switched on when the cells of the body get stressed. In our stressed-out world, we rarely get told that stress is bene-ficial, but in this instance it is. Here we are concerned with a physiological stress acting in a very controlled manner, which causes our body to react and adapt. Sirtuins do this in various ways, such as by increasing the efficiency of muscles, switching on fat burning, reducing inflammation, and repairing and recycling damage and debris that have built up in our cells. By activating this inbuilt 'repair and rejuvenate' programme within our cells, sirtuins help make us fitter, leaner and healthier.

Fasting, exercise and...

Two well-known ways of creating beneficial stress and switching on our sirtuin genes are fasting and exercise. Caloric restriction, a form of fasting that requires a lifelong reduction in calories, has been shown to extend the lifespan of various species. Exercise, as we know, has innumerable health benefits and slashes mortality rates. But as desirable as their sirtuin-activating benefits are, neither is for the faint-hearted when it comes to weight loss.

The word 'hangry' (which if you hadn't already guessed is a mash-up of 'hungry' and 'angry', representing the bad temper and irritability that ensues from feeling famished) has now entered *The Oxford English Dictionary*. Add in fatigue, muscle loss and quite possibly even malnutrition, and fasting rapidly loses its gloss.

When it comes to exercise, as much as we encourage regular moderate amounts for its well-being benefits, it often requires a heroic effort for it to be effective for weight loss. You simply can't outrun a bad diet.

If the effort of fasting or the arduousness of heavy exercise sounds a bit too much like hard work, but you want to get your sirtuin genes working for you, don't despair, as there is a more palatable way, which can be found in the food we eat.

Sirtfoods

Sirtfoods are foods capable of mimicking the effects of fasting and exercise by activating our sirtuin genes, and in so doing enable us to burn fat, build muscle and boost health. Yup, you got it, you get to *eat* your way to great health and a leaner life!

It sounds almost too good to be true, and to really grasp just how foods can do this will require you to think *very* differently about why fruits, vegetables and plant foods are good for you. Up until now, all we've heard is that these foods are good for us largely because of their content of vitamins, minerals, fibre and antioxidants. But we've got a totally different take on this and, if we're being honest, it's one that totally blew our minds when we first came across it. Plant foods are good for us because they are full of weak toxins. Not vitamins. Not minerals. Not antioxidants. Toxins…

WHAT DOESN'T KILL YOU MAKES YOU STRONGER

Natural plant toxins understandably cause stress to our cells, but it is the 'good' kind of stress we mentioned earlier. The type of stress that revs up our sirtuins and causes our cells to adapt and become fitter and healthier. There is a technical name for this phenomenon, which is 'hormesis'. It's an evolutionary survival mechanism, or as we like to say, 'what doesn't kill you makes you stronger'.

Incredibly, all living organisms experience hormesis, including plants. But what's special about plants is just how mind-bogglingly sophisticated their stress response system is compared to our own. And the reason for that is simple: plants are stationary. At first thought that seems really odd, but think about it and you realise that if you are stationary, you're at a massive disadvantage. You can't go in search of water, food or shelter, or flee from an aggressor looking to make dinner from you. You are quite literally rooted to the spot. As a result of this hindrance, plants have developed a dazzlingly high-spec stress response system that helps them adapt to and survive in their environment. It involves producing a vast armamentarium of natural plant chemicals to protect them. These plant chemicals are known as polyphenols.

When we eat these plants, we don't just ingest their vitamins and minerals, we also take in their polyphenols. Effectively, we consume a bunch of highly sophisticated plant stress signals. And guess what? Many of these polyphenols have the ability to activate our own innate stress response pathways. We're talking about exactly the same stress response pathways that are activated by fasting and exercise: the sirtuins. Piggy-backing on a plant's stress response system like this is called xenohormesis and it promises to revolutionise our understanding of why certain foods are good for us. We refer to the foods that are highest in the natural plant compounds that activate sirtuins as 'Sirtfoods'.

GOODBYE FAT

Back when we first trialled the Sirtfood Diet on a group of 40 people, there was one thing that really stood out. It wasn't just the fact that people were losing significant amounts of weight. Rather it was the *type* of weight people were losing that really roused our interest. Typically, when people diet, they lose weight from both fat and muscle. But we saw something very different. People were losing fat without losing muscle. Indeed, much to our surprise, some people actually gained muscle.

That's a big deal for a number of reasons, none more so than losing weight but retaining muscle because it gives that much sought-after toned and lean look. Even better, holding on to muscle means that the drop in metabolic rate that occurs with weight loss is lessened. That muscle keeps on burning energy for you, even when resting. And that helps prevent the dreaded weight regain and stacks the odds in your favour when it comes to keeping the weight off permanently.

To make sense of this shock finding, we need to get back to sirtuins, and a key member of the sirtuin family, Sirt-1, which delivers a triple blow to fat. First, it blocks the action of what's known as PPAR-γ, which orchestrates the process of fat production in the body. Second, it ramps up the activity of what is called PGC-1α which has the really important job of encouraging our cells to make more tiny energy factories that burn fat as fuel. And to top it off, Sirt-1 also coaxes our fat cells to undergo something of a personality change, actually cajoling them to dispose of fat rather than store it.

HELLO MUSCLE

That's a hammer blow to fat, but how to explain the unexpected effects on muscle? It turns out that sirtuins also have major effects on muscle. Indeed, by activating sirtuins it is possible not only to prevent muscle from breaking down but even to promote its regeneration. This is because Sirt-1 boosts very specialised cells within muscle – called satellite cells – which are responsible for muscle growth and renewal.

Indeed, such is the potential benefit to muscle, the activation of Sirt-1 even looks capable of preventing the gradual loss of muscle mass and function that occurs with age. This phenomenon is known as sarcopenia and can really hinder the ability to function well and remain healthy as we get older. This could have a profound effect on our ability to experience rude health and maintain active lives well into old age.

WELLNESS

Stack it all up and activating sirtuins means it's happy days for getting lean for life. But why stop there? There is one other 'side effect' of eating the Sirtfood way, and that is exceptional health that lasts a lifetime.

After all, we're not just fatter as a society, but sicker too, with a sobering 70 per cent of all deaths the result of chronic disease. In spite of all the truly incredible medical advancement, heart disease, cancer, diabetes, dementia and osteoporosis are still disturbingly rife. It's certainly no secret that healthcare systems around the world are buckling under the strain. Yet there is one thing we know for sure, which is that so much of this illness could be prevented with the right dietary approach.

It turns out that a lack of sirtuin activity is implicated in many of these diseases, and activating sirtuins has been shown to have positive effects on the health of the heart and arteries, improve how insulin works in the body, discourage the build-up of damage that leads to dementia, and boost bone-building cells called osteoblasts that help to fend off osteoporosis.

It likely comes as no surprise that a high intake of

processed food, synonymous with our modern-day diet, is linked to reduced sirtuin activity and a high occurrence of chronic disease. But as the Sirtfood Diet brings together the top sirtuin-activating foods that exist, we can now be introduced to a whole world of delicious food and recipes and take comfort knowing that each mouthful sets us up for a lifetime of incredible health.

02

Everything You Need to Know

What do I need?

In terms of equipment, the only essential piece of kit you need is a juicer. In terms of food, the majority of the ingredients will be very familiar and readily available to you. But for Sirtfood Diet first-timers there are a few ingredients about which we want to give you a bit of background.

BUCKWHEAT

In recent times, buckwheat has become the fashionable alternative to grains, driven in no small part by the Sirtfood Diet's success. With influential chefs Jamie Oliver, Nigella Lawson and Lorraine Pascale now embracing this 'pseudo-grain', supermarkets have seen their shelves of buckwheat quickly emptied. The good news is that all this has increased public awareness of buckwheat, with it now being available in its most common forms, groats and flour, in all good supermarkets. When it comes to the 100 per cent buckwheat puffs and flakes you'll find in our recipes, these are still best sourced in healthfood shops or at one of the big online retailers.

MATCHA

Matcha is a concentrated powdered green tea, and what we like to describe as 'green tea on steroids'. It is widely available online and from health food shops, and now starting to appear in supermarkets. There are two things to look out for when it comes to buying matcha. The first is to buy a Japanese version as the alternative Chinese types may be contaminated with heavy metals. The second is to shop around on price. Matcha varies massively in price, with some brands very expensive, but you can find good brands now at very affordable prices.

LOVAGE

This previously overlooked culinary herb is experiencing something of a renaissance since being appointed as a top Sirtfood. If you've never tried it, it tastes like a cross between celery and parsley with hints of curry and aniseed. While it's not yet available in supermarkets (something we hope will soon change), the best place to source it is through your local nursery or online, either as the plant or seeds.

Lovage grows really well in both plant pots and gardens, so all you need is a few seeds, a tray and a windowsill. However, don't despair if you don't have access to it, as you can simply leave it out and still experience the multitude of benefits from all the other Sirtfoods.

CHOCOLATE

Before we leave this section we must also quickly mention everyone's favourite Sirtfood: chocolate! We recommend dark chocolate with 85 per cent cocoa solids, but it is important to note that even at the same cocoa percentage, not all chocolate is equal. Some chocolates go through a refinement process called alkalisation, which greatly reduces their content of sirtuin-activating nutrients. As it is impossible to know from the label which are processed in this way and which are not, we did our own investigating and found that Lindt Excellence 85% Cocoa is not alkalised and is therefore our chocolate of choice. And just in case you thought that darker is necessarily better, their 90% version is alkalised and consequently not as good for you.

The Sirtfood green juice

The green juice is an essential part of Phase 1 of the Sirtfood Diet. All the ingredients are powerful Sirtfoods, and in each juice you get a potent cocktail of natural compounds that work together to turn on your sirtuin genes. All we've added to that is a touch of apple, for taste, and some lemon. Don't overlook the lemon. Its acidic content has been shown to protect, stabilise and increase the absorption of the drink's sirtuin-activating nutrients.

Since publishing *The Sirtfood Diet* book, we have found that fresh ginger really complements the flavours of the juice and brings an invigorating warmth in the mouth. At KX Gym, where the Sirtfood Diet was first trialled, ginger has now replaced apple in the Sirtfood green juice following feedback that it has a more refreshing flavour. So we have included the option to add ginger to this juice as well, either in addition to the apple or to replace it. You can also ignore the ginger altogether and stick with the original tried and trusted recipe if you prefer.

For this book we have also devised some additional juice recipes that you can use to alternate with the classic Sirtfood green juice when you enter Phase 2 and establish Sirtfoods as part of your diet for life (see pages 17–20). After all, variety is the spice of life and we are conscious that no matter how good something is, it can be overdone, and sometimes it is simply good to mix things up.

Before we get to the recipe, the final thing to note is how important it is to make the green juice with a juicer. Unfortunately, high-powered blenders and smoothie makers (such as the Nutribullet) don't work here. We get the appeal;

smoothie makers are convenient, and it seems counter-intuitive that juices are better when they remove all the fibre. When we originally designed the Sirtfood Diet, we were also aboard the smoothie train – until the penny dropped that juicing was the way to go. The reason is that with juicing we can use far more of the leafy green vegetables and get a really concentrated Sirtfood hit in a practical serving. But what about all that roughage that's left behind? When it comes to the desirable sirtuin-activating nutrients, the fibre contains only very small amounts, and we know that too much fibre from leafy greens such as kale can upset our digestive system, especially in sensitive individuals. Thus, on this occasion, it is better to leave it behind.

And we can't leave a juice versus blended discussion without mentioning taste. 'Repungent swamp mix' is one description we heard from someone who initially blended instead of juiced, and we can only agree. Luckily, they have now switched to a juicer and are very much enjoying their tasty and refreshing daily Sirtfood green juice. We also find it interesting to note that when we ran blood tests on our own clients, switching from green smoothies to juices brought about dramatic increases in their levels of other essential nutrients such as magnesium and folic acid. When it comes to juicing versus blending greens, there really is no contest.

Sirtfood green juice (serves 1)

2 large handfuls (75g) kale

a large handful (30g) rocket

a very small handful (5g) flat-leaf parsley

a very small handful (5g) lovage leaves (optional)

2–3 large celery sticks (150g), including leaves

½ medium green apple (optional; it can be replaced by the ginger)

1–2 cm piece of fresh ginger (optional)

juice of ½ lemon

½ level tsp matcha powder*

Note: While in our pilot trial all quantities were weighed out exactly as listed, our experience is that the handful measures work extremely well. In fact, it better tailors the nutrient quantity to an individual's body size. Larger individuals tend to have larger hands and therefore get a proportionally higher amount of Sirtfood nutrients to match their body size and vice versa for smaller people.

• Mix the greens (kale, rocket, parsley and lovage) together, then juice them. We find juicers can really differ in their efficiency at juicing leafy vegetables, and you might need to re-juice the remnants before

* Days 1–3 of Phase 1: added only to the first two juices of the day; days 4–7 of Phase 1: added to both juices

moving on to the other ingredients. The goal is to end up with about 50ml of juice from the greens.

- Now juice the celery and apple or ginger or both.

- You can peel the lemon and put it through the juicer as well, but we find it much easier to simply squeeze the lemon by hand into the juice. By this stage, you should have around 250ml of juice in total, perhaps slightly more.

- It is only when the juice is made and ready to serve that you add the matcha. Pour a small amount of the juice into a glass, then add the matcha and stir vigorously with a fork or teaspoon. We use matcha only in the first two drinks of the day as it contains moderate amounts of caffeine (the same content as a normal cup of tea). For people not used to it, it may keep them awake if drunk late.

- Once the matcha has dissolved, add the remainder of the juice. Give it a final stir and your juice is ready to drink; feel free to top it up with plain water, according to taste.

- You can either make each juice from scratch as and when you want it, or you can make up all your juices for the day in one batch in the morning, and refrigerate until needed, without any loss of potency. In fact, research points to the beneficial sirtuin-activating polyphenols lasting for up to three days before levels start to drop, so if you're short on time, it's perfectly fine to make your juices in advance, ensuring you keep them chilled and away from light.

How to consume your juices

Phase 1, days 1–3: three juices to be drunk daily
Phase 1, days 4–7: two juices to be drunk daily
Phase 2 onwards: one juice to be drunk daily with the option of varying the juice with one of the recipes on pages 234–6.

Who is the diet not suitable for?

While the majority of recipes in this book are suitable for the whole family, there are some important caveats.

Phase 1 of the diet is not suitable for children, anybody trying to conceive or who is pregnant or breastfeeding, and those who are underweight (BMI of less than 18.5).

Individuals with significant health problems, taking

medication, or who have any other reason to be concerned before embarking on the diet, should seek advice from their medical practitioner before starting.

Pregnant women should limit caffeine intake to 200mg max a day (one mug of instant coffee typically contains 100mg of caffeine). They should also avoid matcha altogether and not exceed four cups of regular green tea a day.

The Sirtfood Diet programme is designed for targeting weight loss and is not suitable for children. Likewise, Sirtfoods with noteworthy levels of caffeine (matcha green tea and coffee) should not be given to children. However, that does not mean children can't benefit from including the many other top Sirtfoods in their diet for their exceptional health benefits, as well as enjoying the many recipes in this book that have been created to be family-friendly meals and satisfy taste buds both young and old.

Red wine, despite being a Sirtfood, should only be consumed in moderation due to its alcohol content, and should be avoided completely in pregnancy and, unsurprisingly, not be given to children.

03

Top Tips for Sirt-ain Success

Doing anything for the first time is always a bit daunting, so if you're new to all things Sirt, we want to give you the best possible start. Or maybe you're a Sirtfood Diet veteran, in which case you can use this as an opportunity to ensure you are ticking all the boxes. Either way, after our own trials and errors (of which there were plenty) and the wonderful feedback from all the Sirtfoodies who have been there, done it, and bought the T-shirt, we've put together our top tips for getting the best results from the diet with the minimum of fuss. Follow these and it as good as guaranteed you will hit the ground running on your road to complete success.

1 GET A GOOD JUICER

One of the tenets of the Sirtfood diet is that through juicing the top Sirtfood leafy vegetables we can transform a huge amount of Sirtfood plant material into a simple drink that is perfectly palatable and very easily digested. This means a super-concentrated hit of Sirtfood in a glass.

Of course, to make a juice you need a juicer. While none of us particularly likes splashing out on new kitchen equipment, this is an indispensable bit of kit that you will be using every day to give your well-being a big boost, so we think it's an investment that will reap dividends for your health for years to come. While juicers are largely similar and budget should be the determining factor, people do frequently ask us what juicer we use. We found that some juicers are considerably more effective at extracting the juice from green leafy veg and herbs, with the Sage brand being among the best we have tried.

We must also stress again that while many of us have high-powered blenders and smoothie makers (the Nutribullet and Nutri Ninja spring to mind), these are *not* suitable for making the Sirtfood green juice.

2 PREPARATION IS KEY

Abraham Lincoln famously said, 'Give me six hours to chop down a tree and I will spend the first four sharpening the axe.' Preparation and success go hand in hand, and the Sirtfood Diet is no different. From the many people who have contacted us and shared their experiences, one thing is very clear: those who read and digested the book and planned their first seven days in advance were the most successful.

So as eager as you are to jump straight in, we'd recommend you finish reading the book first. Don't cut corners, and do refer to the book as many times as you need to before getting under way. Get familiar with the recipes you will be following for the week, prepare your shopping list and stock up on all the ingredients and kitchen essentials you'll need. While many of the recipes are quick and easy, don't let that lull you into a false sense of security that you don't need to be prepared. If you know you've a busy day ahead, shop in advance and have all the bases covered. You can even cook a dish or make the juices the night before and store them in the fridge. With everything organised and ready, you'll be amazed at how easy the whole process is.

3 EAT EARLY

When it comes to eating, our philosophy is the earlier the better. This is for two reasons. First, the natural satiating effect of Sirtfoods. There's a lot more benefit to eating a meal that will keep you feeling full, satisfied and energised as you go about your day than spending the whole day feeling hungry only to eat and stay full as you sleep through the night. While the juices do have some natural satiating effects, it is through eating solid food that the benefit of

Sirtfoods shines through, and we found that those who ate their meals earlier in the day reported feeling much fuller and more satisfied than those who waited until night-time. This was particularly true during the first three days of Phase 1, where there is only one meal per day. Those who opted to have their meal at lunchtime generally found it easier than those who waited until dinner.

The second reason is that we all have an inbuilt body clock (called our circadian rhythm) that determines the fate of the food we eat. If we eat earlier in the day, we are more likely to use food as energy, whereas if we eat late in the day, the food is processed differently and more likely to be converted to fat. Because of this, we do suggest you do your best to eat before 7pm each evening, even if it means preparing the next day's meals the night before.

Of course, we live in the real world too and realise that is not always going to be possible for a lot of people. If that's you, and you work late for example, then be flexible with this rule and find a way to make the diet fit around your lifestyle the best you can.

4 EAT UNTIL SATISFIED

One of the key findings from people following the Sirtfood Diet is that the natural satiating effects of Sirtfoods means that some participants found the meals very filling, often being satisfied before finishing them. We thoroughly recommend that you listen to your body and eat until you are comfortably full instead of forcing all the food down to complete the meal just because there is food left on your plate.

While the meals have been designed for typical serving sizes, please remember that we are all different and there is no one-size-fits-all with portion sizes. Once you learn to listen to your internal cues, you can accurately judge for yourself how much is right for you to meet your body's needs. Rather than eat until you are totally stuffed, which never feels great, it might be wiser to take a leaf from the exceptionally long-lived Okinawans, who live by the dictum '*hara hachi bu*', which roughly translates as 'to eat until you are 80 per cent full'.

5 DON'T LET THE SCALES DICTATE

In our original pilot study the average weight loss over seven days, after adjusting for muscle gain, was 7lb (3.2kg). While that was the average, there was actually a lot of variation between people, with weight loss on the scales varying all the way from 3lb (1.4kg) to over 10lb (4.5kg). Did this mean that those who lost the most weight were the most successful, and those who lost the least were failures? Not at all!

As much as people are hooked on the idea that the scales are the ultimate judge of our success, we would encourage you to think differently, especially if what you are really after is lasting weight loss and a lifetime of great health. There are two things that are actually far more important. The first is to lose the right *type* of fat. That might sound odd, but where we store fat is very important and some fat is much more harmful than others. Here we're talking about the fat that accumulates around the tummy area. This type of 'central adiposity' is strongly linked to major metabolic diseases, such as diabetes and heart disease for example.

The second is to maintain or even increase muscle mass. Not only does this give a desirable lean, toned and athletic look, but it also keeps your metabolism high, as muscle is constantly burning up energy for you, even at rest. This really helps to further support weight loss and increases the likelihood of success in the long term.

With the Sirtfood Diet both of these outcomes are not only achievable but very common. In fact we often see the scales creeping up in the last few days of Phase 1 due to muscle gain, while waistlines continue to shrink. That's why we want you to look at the scales, but not be ruled by them. Check out how you look in the mirror, how your clothes are fitting or whether you need to move a notch on your belt. These are all great indicators of the more profound changes in your body composition. And remember, weight loss aside, the introduction of Sirtfoods into your diet is a huge step in making your cells fitter and more resistant to disease, setting you up for a lifetime of exceptional health.

6 ENJOY THE JOURNEY

The beauty of the Sirtfood Diet is that it is a diet of inclusion. It's all about introducing great foods into your diet. Some of them may be new, others you simply might not have thought to include in the quantities we recommend.

It's not about eating for the sake of eating or just grinning and bearing it because you think it is doing you good. This diet is about celebrating food in all its wonder, for its health benefits but equally for the pleasure and enjoyment it brings.

So many diets are nothing more than a means to an end, based on the premise of 'no pain, no gain' and assuming that we must endure hardship and deprivation to get results. The Sirtfood Diet puts an end to that fallacy. In fact, what a shame it would be if we were so focused on achieving our weight-loss targets that we didn't stop to appreciate all the amazing foods and delicious recipes along the way.

It's all about being mindful and appreciating the here and now. This is actually backed up by research too, which shows that when we keep our mind focused on the path instead of the final destination we are much more likely to succeed. So, enjoy the moment and every delicious mouthful it brings.

7 DON'T BE AFRAID TO EXPERIMENT

While the recipes in this book have been designed by one of Britain's highly talented chefs and bring an explosion of taste even to the quickest and simplest of meals, please feel free to be creative. There's nothing more we love to see than our readers going freestyle and adding their own personal flair to their Sirtfood experience. Whether it's to tweak a recipe because of a dietary restriction, or because you're a spice fiend who demands chilli with *everything* (we've heard from people who are adding chilli to their Sirtfood juices!), or simply just to make it more 'you', we say go for it. Or perhaps you'll use a recipe as a starting point or inspiration for your own Sirtified masterpiece? Nothing would make us happier and we love hearing about your culinary adventures. The greatest outcome we can achieve with this book is for you to fully embrace the benefits of Sirtfoods to the point where you instinctively begin to 'Sirtify' your normal dietary habits. At that point, eating Sirtfoods becomes second nature and a way of eating for life.

8 ENGAGE IN MODERATE PHYSICAL ACTIVITY

Besides what we eat, engaging in exercise is the best thing we can do for our health. It brings a whole constellation of benefits to both body and mind, and its positive effects are incredibly well studied. Although many of the benefits of exercise are brought about through activating our sirtuin genes, adding exercise to a Sirtfood-rich diet can really max out sirtuin activation.

During Phase 1 of the diet we recommend you curtail exercise efforts to a comfortable level as you will be relying on mild fasting to give you that maximum sirtuin bang. But after that you can exercise freely according to your personal preference in the knowledge that the combination of exercise and a Sirtfood-rich diet offers the perfect pairing for both enhancing your exercise performance and recovery, while boosting weight loss and health. As a minimum, we strongly urge you to meet government guidelines of 30 minutes of moderate physical activity – brisk walking, jogging or going to the gym – on five days a week.

9 THE FIBRE FACTOR

Many Sirtfoods are naturally rich in fibre – onions, chicory and walnuts being notable sources. But it is buckwheat and Medjool dates that really stand out as having a high fibre content. During days 1–3 of Phase 1, where only one meal is consumed each day, alongside three green juices (from which the fibre is removed to allow for more sirtuin-activating ingredients to be concentrated in the juice), some of us will need to be conscious that our meal selection is high in fibre to maintain gut regularity and avoid constipation. This can really vary from one person to another, but if you feel you need a fibre boost, make a conscious effort to select recipes that contain buckwheat, beans, chickpeas or lentils.

10 DRINK UP

It's likely you've heard the advice that we need to drink eight glasses of water a day to stay hydrated. Or the idea that if we feel thirsty the body is already dehydrated. Neither claim has any real scientific basis. But there are still real advantages to regular fluid intake, especially as by choosing the right beverages you can ramp up your intake of Sirtfood goodness in a way that's really convenient, tasty and can be done just as easily whether you are at home, at work or out with friends. The green juice is one obvious way to really boost Sirtfood intake. But remember that both green tea and coffee are top Sirtfoods. And contrary to the popular myth that caffeine dehydrates the body, green tea and coffee both count towards your daily fluid intake if consumed regularly. White tea and black tea are also good Sirtfood options. And why not jazz up still or sparkling water in both taste and nutritional quality by adding some sliced strawberries to make your own Sirtfood-infused health drink?

Recipes

Recipe notes

Before you get stuck into the recipes, we've just a few notes to share, to make sure you hit the ground running.

- Bird's eye chillies (sometimes sold as 'Thai chillies') are one of the top 20 Sirtfoods and appear regularly throughout these recipes. If you have never tried them, they are notably hotter than normal chillies. If you are not used to spicy food, we suggest starting off with half the chilli amount stated in the recipe, as well as deseeding your chilli before use. From here you can adjust the heat to your preference throughout the diet.
- If you haven't cooked buckwheat before, it couldn't be easier. We recommend that you first wash the buckwheat thoroughly in a sieve before placing it in a pan of boiling water. Cooking times can vary, so do check the instructions on your packet.

- Miso is a delicious, flavour-packed, fermented soya bean paste. You will find it comes in a range of colours, typically white, yellow, red and brown. The lighter-coloured miso pastes are sweeter than the dark ones, which can be quite salty. For our recipes, brown or red miso will work well, but by all means experiment and see which flavours you prefer. Red miso tends to be the saltier of the two, so if you do opt for this one, you might prefer to use a little less of it. The flavour and saltiness of miso can also vary between brands so that the best bet would be to check whatever type you buy and adjust the amount you use accordingly so that it's not too overpowering. That means a little trial and error, but you'll soon get the hang of it.
- Capers can vary in size. For our recipes, the smaller ones (nonpareille capers) work best but if you can only get larger ones, this is perfectly fine – all you need to do is chop them to the desired size and consistency.
- Flat-leaf parsley would be best for all the dishes, but if you can't get hold of it, the curly variety will do.
- Onions, garlic and ginger are always peeled unless otherwise stated.
- Salt and pepper are not used in these recipes but feel free to season with sea salt and black pepper according to your preferences. Sirtfoods offer so much flavour that you will likely find you do not need as much seasoning as you would normally use.

Recipe labelling

To help you select the recipes that best fit your dietary requirements, we've developed a simple labelling system to guide you on each recipe, as follows:

 Vegetarian

 Vegan

 Dairy free

 Gluten free

 Quick and easy

 Batch cook

Note that recipes marked as gluten free contain naturally gluten-free ingredients, but for some products there is a risk of cross-contamination with gluten, so those following a strict gluten-free diet should refer to product labels for assurances.

So that's it! You're bang up to date with Sirtfoods and how to succeed. That just leaves you to get cracking with all the mouth-watering recipes this book contains. Happy eating!

Days 1–3

Phase 1 is a serious kick-start to weight loss and great health. It's what we call the 'hyper-success' phase and is the proven method for losing 7lb (3.2kg) in seven days.

The reason it's so successful is because it combines moderate fasting with a diet packed to the rafters with Sirtfoods – in short, a powerful two-pronged approach that fires up your sirtuin genes.

Phase 1 lasts for just seven days, and has two distinct stages. This chapter takes you through the first three days, which is the most intensive stage. Over the three days you can consume up to 1,000 calories each day, which will consist of:

- 3 x Sirtfood green juices (see page 35)
- 1 x main meal
- 15–20g dark chocolate (85 per cent cocoa solids)

It is best to spread the green juices out over the day. So for example, you might take one first thing in the morning, one mid morning, and another mid afternoon. To be most effective, they should be consumed at least an hour before or two hours after the meal.

When it comes to the main meal, you are free to choose from any of the recipes in this chapter. It's done on a pick 'n' mix basis, which leaves you complete freedom to choose the recipes that fit your tastes, dietary preferences and lifestyle. Gluten-free, dairy-free, vegetarian and vegan options are all well catered for. Likewise, we've included a good smattering of quick and easy options for those for whom time is a scarce commodity.

All these options are labelled in the recipes for ease of reference, so go with whatever recipes work for you. The only rule is to choose a different one on each of the three days, which helps to ensure you are getting a full spectrum of Sirtfoods.

In the spirit of saving the best until last, you get to eat chocolate from day one, so it's happy days from the get-go. Most people have their 15–20g of 85 per cent dark chocolate as a mini dessert after their main meal.

As well as the three green juices, you can consume other fluids freely throughout Phase 1. Drinks should be non-caloric and preferably plain water, black coffee or green tea. Red wine is not introduced until week two. The one thing we don't recommend, however, is a sudden large change to your normal coffee/caffeine consumption, as both sudden increases and decreases can leave you feeling lousy.

Grilled green tea and chicken kebabs with rocket and chickpea salad

SERVES 1

1 medium chicken breast, cut into chunks
60g red onion, cut into chunks
1 level tsp matcha
1 tsp extra virgin olive oil
juice of ¼ – ½ lemon, depending on taste
1 garlic clove, finely chopped
1cm piece of fresh ginger, finely chopped
1 tsp tamari (or soy sauce if not avoiding gluten)

For the salad

30g rocket
50g carrot, grated
40g celery, finely sliced
35g chickpeas
juice of ½ lemon
1 tsp tamari (or soy sauce if not avoiding gluten)
1 tsp extra virgin olive oil
1 tsp sesame seeds
1cm piece of fresh ginger, very finely grated

Combine all the kebab ingredients in a bowl and set aside to marinate. The longer you can leave the chicken the better – 1 hour would be ideal, but if you give it only 10 minutes while you prepare the other elements, it will still pack a punch.

If you are using wooden skewers, soak them now in a little water. Heat your grill on its highest setting.

Meanwhile, prepare the salad. In a bowl, mix the rocket, carrot, celery and chickpeas. For the dressing mix the lemon juice with the remaining ingredients. Pour the dressing over the salad and mix well.

Thread the chicken and red onion on to your skewers and grill for 8–10 minutes, turning them over halfway through the cooking. Serve with the dressed salad.

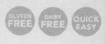

Miso-marinated turkey escalope with chilli salsa and buckwheat

If you can find only turkey steak, there are two ways to turn it into an escalope. Depending on how thick the steak is, you can either use a meat tenderiser, hammer or a rolling pin to bash it until it is around 5mm thick. Or, if you feel the steak is too thick for this to work, and you have a steady hand, cut the steak in half horizontally and then bash each piece with the tenderiser.

SERVES 1

20g red miso
1 tsp mirin
1 tsp extra virgin olive oil
125–150g turkey escalope or turkey breast steak
1 tbsp ground turmeric
50g buckwheat

For the salsa

130g tomato
10g red onion
1 tsp capers

1 bird's eye chilli
juice of ½ lemon
1 tbsp chopped parsley
1 tsp extra virgin olive oil

Mix the miso, mirin and olive oil together and rub the mixture into the escalope. Ideally, you should leave this to marinate for 1 hour, but if you want to use it straight away, you can.

Heat your grill on its highest setting.

Place 500ml of water in a saucepan with the turmeric, bring to the boil and cook the buckwheat as directed on your packet. Drain and reserve.

Meanwhile, prepare the salsa. Finely chop the tomato, red onion, capers and chilli, making sure you keep all the liquid from the tomato. Mix with the lemon juice, parsley and oil.

Grill the turkey for 5 minutes on each side, watching it carefully so as not to burn the marinade. Serve with the salsa and buckwheat.

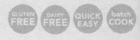

Prawn arrabbiata with buckwheat pasta

The tomato-based sauce below also works really well for the Sirt shakshuka recipe on page 92. To save time make double and keep half in the fridge for up to three days to have when you need it.

SERVES 1

65g buckwheat pasta
1 tsp olive oil
125–150g raw or cooked prawns (ideally king prawns)

For the arrabbiata sauce

40g red onion, finely chopped
1 garlic clove, finely chopped
30g celery, finely chopped
1 bird's-eye chilli, finely chopped
1 tsp herbes de Provence or dried mixed herbs
1 tsp extra virgin olive oil
2 tbsp white wine (optional)
1 x 400g tin of chopped tomatoes
1 tbsp chopped parsley

First make the sauce. Fry the onion, garlic, celery, chilli and dried herbs in the oil over a medium–low heat for 1–2 minutes. Turn the heat up to medium, add the wine (if using) and cook for 1 minute. Add the tomatoes and leave the sauce to simmer over a medium–low heat for 20–30 minutes, until it has a nice rich consistency. If you feel the sauce is getting too thick, simply add a little water.

While the sauce is cooking, bring a large pan of water to the boil and cook the pasta according to the packet instructions. When ready, drain, toss with the olive oil and keep in the pan until needed.

If you are using raw prawns, add them to the sauce and cook for a further 3–4 minutes, until they have turned pink and opaque, then add the parsley. If you are using cooked prawns, add them with the parsley and bring the sauce to the boil.

Add the cooked pasta to the sauce, mix thoroughly but gently and serve.

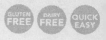

Sirt moules marinière

SERVES 1

300g live mussels
50g buckwheat
30g kale, roughly chopped
40g red onion, finely chopped
40g celery, finely chopped
2 garlic cloves, finely chopped
2 tbsp chopped parsley
100ml white wine
1 tbsp extra virgin olive oil

To prepare the mussels, remove their beards. This is a stringy membrane that can simply be pulled off. Tap each mussel gently and discard any that do not close as these are dead. Place the mussels in a colander and rinse under running water to remove any bits of grit. If possible, try to use your mussels on the day of purchase to maximise freshness.

Place 750ml of water in a saucepan, bring to the boil and cook the buckwheat according to the packet instructions, adding the kale for the last 5 minutes of the cooking time. Drain and set aside.

Place a large saucepan that has a lid over a high heat, until it starts to smoke. Add the cleaned mussels – they will hiss and spit but this is perfectly fine. Immediately add the red onion, celery, garlic, parsley and wine. Mix thoroughly and place a lid on top of the pan to steam the mussels, keeping them over a high heat.

The mussels will cook very quickly and should be ready in 2–3 minutes, at which point they should all have opened (discard any that haven't). Stir them every 30 seconds or so to regulate the heat within the pan. Be careful not to overcook them as they become tough and tasteless. Stir through the olive oil, buckwheat and kale and serve.

Turmeric-baked salmon with spicy celery

SERVES 1

1 tsp ground turmeric
1 tsp extra virgin olive oil
juice of ¼ lemon
125–150g skinned salmon fillet

For the spicy celery

1 tsp extra virgin olive oil
40g red onion, finely chopped
1 garlic clove, finely chopped
1cm piece of fresh ginger, finely chopped
1 bird's-eye chilli, finely chopped
150g celery, cut into 2cm pieces
1 tsp mild curry powder
130g (about 1) tomato, cut into 8 wedges
100ml chicken or vegetable stock
60g tinned green lentils, drained and rinsed
1 tbsp chopped parsley

Heat the oven to 200°C/Gas 6.

Start with the spicy celery. Heat a frying pan over a medium–low heat, add the olive oil, then the onion, garlic, ginger, chilli and celery. Fry gently for 2–3 minutes, or until softened but not coloured, then add the curry powder and cook for a further minute.

Add the tomato then the stock and lentils and simmer gently for 10 minutes. You may want to increase or decrease the cooking time, depending on how crunchy you like your celery.

Meanwhile, mix the turmeric, oil and lemon juice and rub over the salmon. Place on a baking tray and cook for 8–10 minutes

To finish, stir the parsley through the celery and serve with the salmon.

Stir-fried pork fillet with kale and walnuts

You could swap the pork for beef fillet or the equivalent weight of chicken breast if you'd prefer.

SERVES 1

125–150g pork fillet
1 tsp extra virgin olive oil
juice of ¼ lemon
1 tsp ground turmeric

For the buckwheat

1 tbsp ground turmeric
50g buckwheat

For the vegetables

1 tsp extra virgin olive oil
40g red onion, finely chopped
1 garlic clove, finely chopped
1 bird's-eye chilli, finely chopped
1cm piece of fresh ginger, finely chopped

1 tsp ground cumin

50g kale, roughly chopped

20g green beans, cut in half

20g celery, thinly sliced

100ml chicken stock

1 tsp tamari (or soy sauce if not avoiding gluten)

20g chopped walnuts

1 tbsp chopped coriander

First make the buckwheat: put 500ml of cold water into a saucepan, add the turmeric and bring to the boil. Cook the buckwheat according to the packet instructions and set aside until needed.

Trim any fat from the pork and cut it into 1cm-thick slices. Mix with the olive oil, lemon juice and turmeric. Heat a frying pan over a medium–high heat, add the pork and stir-fry for 3–4 minutes, until cooked through, then remove from the pan and set aside on plate.

Place the olive oil for the vegetables in the frying pan over a low heat. Add the red onion, garlic, chilli and ginger and when softened but not coloured, add the cumin and cook for a further minute.

Add the kale, green beans and celery and cook gently for 2–3 minutes, then add the stock and tamari. Cook for a further couple of minutes over a low–medium heat or until the vegetables are tender. Add the walnuts, coriander and the cooked pork, mix well and serve with the buckwheat.

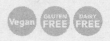

Spiced chickpeas with butternut squash, dates and walnuts

SERVES 1

2 large Medjool dates, pitted and chopped

100ml hot vegetable stock

100g butternut squash

1 tsp extra virgin olive oil

40g red onion, sliced

1 bird's eye chilli, finely chopped

1 garlic clove, finely chopped

1 tsp ground turmeric

1 tsp paprika

½ tsp ground cinnamon

1 tsp ground cumin

150g tinned chickpeas, drained and rinsed

20g chopped walnuts

1 tbsp chopped parsley

15g rocket

Place the chopped dates in the hot stock and set aside until required.

Peel the butternut squash and cut into bite-sized chunks. Place in a pan of boiling water and leave to simmer for 10–15 minutes – watch it carefully as you don't want it to go mushy. Drain and set aside.

Heat a saucepan or casserole over a low heat, add the olive oil, onion, chilli and garlic and fry gently for 2 minutes. Add the turmeric, paprika, cinnamon and cumin and cook for a further minute or so.

Add the chickpeas, walnuts and date/stock mixture and bring to the boil. Cook for a minute, then add the squash and parsley.

Just before you are ready to serve, remove the pan from the heat and stir through the rocket.

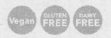

Kale, coconut and tofu Thai curry

SERVES 1

100ml vegetable stock
1 tsp tamari (or soy sauce if not avoiding gluten)
150ml coconut milk
50g kale, roughly chopped
30g carrot, roughly chopped
30g celery, roughly chopped
150g firm tofu, cut into 2cm dice
6–8 basil leaves

For the curry paste

30g red onion, roughly chopped
1cm piece of fresh ginger, roughly chopped
1 garlic clove, roughly chopped
1 bird's eye chilli, roughly chopped
1 lemongrass stalk, bashed then roughly chopped
1 tbsp chopped parsley
1 tsp ground turmeric
1 tsp ground cumin
1 tsp extra virgin olive oil

For the buckwheat

1tbsp ground turmeric
50g buckwheat

Place all the ingredients for the paste in a blender and blend until you have a fine paste.

Transfer the paste to a saucepan and cook it gently over a low heat for 2–3 minutes. Add the stock, tamari and the coconut milk and cook for 20 minutes.

Meanwhile, put 500ml of cold water into a saucepan, add the turmeric and bring to the boil. Cook the buckwheat according to the packet instructions and set aside until needed.

Add the kale, carrot and celery to the curry and cook for a further 10 minutes. Stir in the tofu and basil, bring to the boil, then immediately remove from the heat and serve with the cooked buckwheat.

Buckwheat pasta with Sirt arrabbiata sauce

The tomato-based sauce below works really well for the Sirt shakshuka recipe on page 92. To save time make double and keep half in the fridge for up to three days to have when you need it.

SERVES 1

40g red onion, finely chopped
1 garlic clove, finely chopped
30g celery, finely chopped
1 bird's eye chilli, finely chopped
2 tsp extra virgin olive oil
1 tsp herbes de Provence or dried mixed herbs
1 tbsp white wine (optional)
1 x 400g tin of chopped tomatoes
40g kale, roughly chopped
1 tbsp chopped parsley
1 tsp capers
75g buckwheat pasta
1 tbsp pine nuts, toasted

Fry the onion, garlic, celery and chilli in 1 teaspoon of the oil with the dried herbs over a medium–low heat for 1–2 minutes. Turn the heat up to medium, add the wine (if using) and cook for 1 minute. Add the tomatoes and leave the sauce to simmer over a medium–low heat for 20 minutes, then add the kale and cook for a further 10 minutes. If you feel the sauce is getting too thick, simply add a little water. When the sauce has a nice rich consistency, stir in the parsley and capers.

While the sauce is cooking, bring a pan of water to the boil and cook the pasta according to the packet instructions. When ready, drain, toss with the olive oil and keep in the pan until needed.

Add the cooked pasta to the sauce, mix thoroughly but gently and serve with the pine nuts scattered over the top.

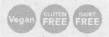

Stir-fried noodles with chilli and miso

SERVES 1

75g buckwheat noodles
2 tsp extra virgin olive oil
5g dried arame
25g miso paste
40g red onion, thinly sliced
40g celery, thinly sliced
1 garlic clove, finely chopped
1cm piece of fresh ginger, finely chopped
1 bird's eye chilli, finely chopped
50g carrot, grated
30g mushrooms, sliced
50g kale, roughly chopped
1 tbsp chopped coriander

Cook the noodles according to the packet instructions.
When ready, drain, mix with 1 teaspoon of the olive oil
and set aside until needed.

Cover the arame with boiling water, leave for 5 minutes, then drain. Mix 100ml of boiling water with the miso paste and stir until dissolved.

Heat the remaining teaspoon of olive oil in a frying pan, add the onion, celery, garlic, ginger and chilli and fry over a low–medium heat for 1–2 minutes.

Add the carrot, mushrooms and kale, increase the heat to medium and cook for 2–3 minutes.

Toss in the noodles and continue to cook for a minute or so, continually stirring so that the noodles don't stick. Add the miso broth, bring to the boil, then remove from the heat and leave to stand for 1 minute – the noodles should absorb most of the remaining liquid. Stir through the chopped coriander and arame and serve.

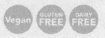

Braised Puy lentils with kale and slow-roasted cherry tomatoes

SERVES 1

8 cherry tomatoes, halved
2 tsp extra virgin olive oil
40g red onion, thinly sliced
1 garlic clove, finely chopped
40g celery, thinly sliced
40g carrot, thinly sliced
1 tsp paprika
1 tsp thyme (dried or fresh)
75g dried Puy lentils
220ml vegetable stock
50g kale, roughly chopped
1 tbsp chopped parsley
20g rocket

Heat your oven to 120°C/gas ½.

Put the tomatoes into a small roasting tin and roast in the oven for 35–45 minutes.

Heat a saucepan over a low–medium heat. Add 1 teaspoon of the olive oil with the red onion, garlic, celery and carrot and fry for 1–2 minutes, until softened. Stir in the paprika and thyme and cook for a further minute.

Rinse the lentils in a fine-meshed sieve and add them to the pan along with the stock. Bring to the boil, then reduce the heat and simmer gently for 20 minutes with a lid on the pan. Give the pan a stir every 7 minutes or so, adding a little water if the level drops too much.

Add the kale and cook for a further 10 minutes. When the lentils are cooked, stir in the parsley and roasted tomatoes. Serve with the rocket drizzled with the remaining teaspoon of olive oil.

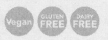

Green tea tofu kebab with rocket and seaweed salad

SERVES 1

150g firm tofu, cut into chunks
60g red onion, cut into chunks
1 level tsp matcha green tea
1 tsp extra virgin olive oil
juice of ¼ – ½ lemon depending on preference
1 garlic clove, finely chopped
1cm piece of fresh ginger, finely chopped
1 tsp tamari (or soy sauce if not avoiding gluten)

For the salad

7g arame
juice of ½ lime
1 tsp tamari (or soy sauce if not avoiding gluten)
1 tsp extra virgin olive oil
1 tsp sesame seeds
1cm piece of fresh ginger, finely grated
50g carrot, grated
40g celery, thinly sliced
40g rocket

Mix the tofu and red onion with all the remaining ingredients for the kebab. The longer you can marinate the tofu the better, ideally 1 hour, but if you can only give it 10 minutes while you prepare the other elements, it will still pack a punch.

If you are using wooden skewers soak them now in a little water. Heat your grill on its highest setting.

Place the arame in a bowl and cover with boiling water. Leave for 5 minutes, then drain and dry thoroughly.

For the dressing mix the lime juice, tamari, olive oil and sesame seeds. Grate the ginger as finely as possible into the mixture.

Thread the tofu and red onion on to your skewers, then grill for 8–10 minutes, turning them halfway through the cooking.

Mix the carrot, celery and rocket for the salad. When your kebabs are ready toss the dressing through the salad and serve.

PHASE 1:

Days 4–7

With the first three days of Phase 1 under your belt, you are well on your way to Sirtfood success. In fact, that's the hardest part done as for the next four days you'll be upping your food intake. You'll do this by dropping one of the green juices and adding in a second daily meal. Over the four-day period you can eat up to 1,500 calories each day, which will consist of:

- 2 x Sirtfood green juices (see page 35)
- 2 x main meals

When it comes to the green juices, it's still good to spread them over the day. Now you are down to two, we would suggest you take one either first thing in the morning or mid-morning, and the other one mid-afternoon. As before, they should be consumed at least an hour before or two hours after the meal.

The good news is that you now get to tuck into two delicious Sirtfood-packed meals each day. The most common way to do this is to eat the first meal during the daytime and the second for dinner in the evening, but be flexible and fit it around what works for you.

The daytime meal can be eaten for breakfast, brunch or lunch, whatever works for you. All you need to do is select any meal from the 'Meal 1' section of this chapter and eat it whenever works best for you.

For dinner simply select any meal from the 'Meal 2' section of this chapter.

MEAL 1

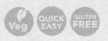

Date and walnut buckwheat porridge with strawberries

For added Sirt goodness you could stir 1 teaspoon of cocoa powder or 1 teaspoon of ground turmeric into the milk.

SERVES 1

200ml milk or dairy-free alternative
1 Medjool date, chopped
35g buckwheat flakes
1 tsp walnut butter or 4 chopped walnut halves
50g strawberries, hulled

Place the milk and date in a pan, heat gently, then add the buckwheat flakes and cook until the porridge is your desired consistency.

Stir in the walnut butter or walnuts, top with the strawberries and serve.

Sirt shakshuka (baked eggs with spicy tomato sauce and kale)

While the sauce here is not quite the same as the Sirt arrabbiata from days 1–3 (see page 77), the two are similar so it also works very well in this recipe and saves a lot of time if you have already made a batch. If you are making the shakshuka from scratch, try making the sauce the night before to save time in the morning.

A small, deep-sided frying pan is ideal for this recipe. The shakshuka is best eaten directly from the pan.

SERVES 1

1 tsp extra virgin olive oil
40g red onion, finely chopped
1 garlic clove, finely chopped
30g celery, finely chopped
1 bird's eye chilli, finely chopped
1 tsp ground cumin
1 tsp ground turmeric
1 tsp paprika
1 x 400g tin of chopped tomatoes
30g kale, stalks removed, roughly chopped

1 tbsp chopped parsley
2 medium eggs

Heat a small, deep-sided frying pan over a medium–low heat. Add the oil and fry the onion, garlic, celery, chilli and spices for 1–2 minutes.

Add the tomatoes, then leave the sauce to simmer gently for 20 minutes, stirring occasionally.

Add the kale and cook for a further 5 minutes. If you feel the sauce is getting too thick, simply add a little water. When your sauce has a nice rich consistency, stir in the parsley.

Make two little wells in the sauce and crack each egg into them. Reduce the heat to its lowest setting and cover the pan with a lid or foil. Leave the eggs to cook for 10–12 minutes, at which point the whites should be firm while the yolks are still runny. Cook for a further 3–4 minutes if you prefer the yolks to be firm. Serve immediately – ideally straight from the pan.

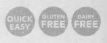

Rocket and smoked salmon omelette

SERVES 1

2 medium eggs
100g smoked salmon, sliced
½ tsp capers
10g rocket, chopped
1 tsp chopped parsley
1 tsp extra virgin olive oil

Crack the eggs into a bowl and whisk well. Add the salmon, capers, rocket and parsley.

Heat the olive oil in a non-stick frying pan until hot but not smoking. Add the egg mixture and, using a spatula or fish slice, move the mixture around the pan until it is even. Reduce the heat and let the omelette cook through. Slide the spatula around the edges and roll up or fold the omelette in half to serve.

Chicken, avocado, rocket and buckwheat crackers

SERVES 1

½ avocado
juice of ¼ lemon
1 tsp extra virgin olive oil
20g celery, diced
20g red onion, diced
100g cooked chicken breast, cut into bite-sized pieces
2–3 buckwheat crackers (shop-bought or home-made see
   page 193)
10g rocket

Peel and stone the avocado, then mash with the back of
a fork. Add the lemon juice, olive oil, celery and red
onion and mix well.

Stir in the chicken. Spread the mixture over the crackers
and top with the rocket.

Buckwheat gallo pinto (fried eggs with spiced buckwheat and beans)

This is a perfect way to use up any leftover buckwheat for a delicious take on a Costa Rican classic.

SERVES 1

2 tsp extra virgin olive oil
30g red onion, diced
30g celery, diced
15g kale (weight with stalks removed), chopped
1 bird's eye chilli, chopped
1 tsp paprika
1 tsp ground turmeric
60g cooked buckwheat
50g tinned black beans or kidney beans, drained and rinsed
1 tbsp chopped coriander
2 medium eggs

Place a small saucepan over a low–medium heat. Add 1 teaspoon of the olive oil and fry the red onion, celery, kale and chilli for 2–3 minutes or until softened. Add the spices and cook for a further minute.

Add the buckwheat, beans and a splash of water and allow them to heat through. Add the coriander.

Meanwhile, prepare the eggs. Place a frying pan over a medium heat, add the remaining teaspoon of olive oil and fry the eggs to your liking. Serve over the buckwheat and beans.

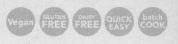

Chilli and turmeric hummus

This is delicious served with celery sticks and home-made buckwheat and seed crackers (see page 193). You could also try leaving out the turmeric and chilli and adding 5g of chopped parsley, 10g of chopped rocket and 1 teaspoon of capers in their place.

SERVES 2

1 x 400g tin of chickpeas, drained and rinsed
2 tbsp tahini
1 tbsp extra virgin olive oil
juice of 1 lemon
50ml water
1 bird's eye chilli, chopped
1 tsp ground turmeric

Place all the ingredients in a food processor and blitz for 2–3 minutes, until you have a smooth paste. You might want to add some more water, depending on how thick you like your hummus.

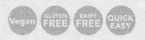

Scrambled tofu with kale, red onion and tomato

SERVES 1

100g extra firm tofu

30g kale (weight with stalks removed), chopped

1 tsp ground turmeric

1 tsp extra virgin olive oil

20g red onion, sliced

20g celery, sliced

½ bird's eye chilli, sliced

5 cherry tomatoes, halved

5g parsley, chopped

Wrap the tofu in kitchen paper and place something heavy on top to help remove any excess water. Steam the kale for 2–3 minutes

Mix the turmeric and a little water until you have a light paste.

Place a frying pan over a medium heat, add the olive oil, then the onion, celery and chilli and fry for 2–3 minutes.

Crumble the tofu into bite-sized pieces and add it to the pan along with the cherry tomatoes, then pour over the turmeric paste and mix thoroughly. Add the kale and continue to stir and fry until the tofu is browned. Toss in the parsley and serve.

Smoked trout, cottage cheese and caper crackers

SERVES 1

50g cottage cheese
1 tsp capers
1 tsp chopped parsley
20g red onion, diced
2–3 buckwheat crackers (shop-bought or home-made see
   page 193)
10g rocket
75g smoked trout, sliced
squeeze of lemon juice

Mix the cottage cheese, capers, parsley and red onion together in a bowl.

Spread the mixture on to the crackers and top with the rocket and smoked trout. Squeeze over the lemon juice to serve.

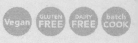

Kale and toasted walnut soup

Most people find this soup filling enough on its own, but you can serve it with home-made buckwheat and seed crackers (see page 193) if you wish.

SERVES 1

2 tsp extra virgin olive oil
30g red onion, sliced
30g celery, sliced
1 garlic clove, sliced
1 tsp dried thyme
75g tinned or home-cooked white beans, such as cannellini
  or haricot
500ml vegetable stock
50g kale, roughly chopped
4 walnut halves, chopped

In a medium saucepan, heat 1 teaspoon of the olive oil over a low–medium heat and fry the red onion, celery and garlic for 2–3 minutes. When they have softened, add the thyme, beans and stock and bring to the boil.

Simmer for 25 minutes over a low heat, then add the kale and cook for a further 10 minutes. When all the vegetables are cooked through, blend the mixture until smooth. You might have to add a little water if your soup is too thick. If it looks very watery before you blend it, simply increase the heat and leave it to bubble until it is thicker.

While the soup is cooking, heat your oven to 160°C/gas 3 and toast your walnuts for 10–15 minutes so that they are nicely browned – watch them carefully as they can easily go from toasted to burnt.

Serve your soup drizzled with the remaining teaspoon of olive oil and topped with the toasted walnuts.

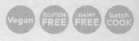

Spicy lentil and vegetable soup

Most people find this soup filling enough on its own, but you can serve it with home-made buckwheat crackers (see page 193) if you wish.

SERVES 1

1 tsp extra virgin olive oil, plus extra for drizzling
30g red onion, diced
30g celery, diced
30g carrot, diced
1 bird's eye chilli, chopped
1 garlic clove, chopped
1 tsp ground turmeric
1 tsp curry powder
500ml vegetable stock
50g red lentils
1 tsp chopped parsley

In a small saucepan, heat the olive oil over a low–medium heat and fry the onion, celery and carrot for 2–3 minutes until they have started to soften. Add the chilli, garlic and spices and cook for a further minute.

Add the vegetable stock and lentils and bring to the boil. Simmer gently for 30 minutes, stirring from time to time to ensure nothing sticks to the bottom.

Once the lentils have broken down and you have a nice soupy consistency, stir through the parsley and serve with a drizzle of extra virgin olive oil.

Sirt coronation chicken salad

SERVES 1

75g natural yoghurt

juice of ¼ lemon

1 tsp chopped coriander

1 tsp ground turmeric

½ tsp mild curry powder

100g cooked chicken breast, cut into bite-sized pieces

6 walnut halves, chopped

1 Medjool date, finely chopped

20g red onion, diced

1 bird's eye chilli

40g rocket, to serve

Mix the yoghurt, lemon juice, coriander and spices together in a bowl. Add all the remaining ingredients and serve on a bed of the rocket.

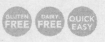

Tuna and chicory boats

SERVES 1

1 x 150g tin of tuna (in oil or brine), drained
20g red onion, diced
20g celery, diced
1 tsp capers
1 tsp chopped parsley
juice of ¼ lemon
1 tsp extra virgin olive oil
1 head of chicory
5–6 walnut halves, chopped

Place the tuna a bowl and add the onion, celery, capers, parsley, lemon juice and olive oil. Mix well.

Slice the end off the chicory head and separate the leaves. Spoon the tuna into as many of the leaves as possible and scatter over the chopped walnuts.

Kale, red onion and cheese frittata

A small, deep-sided non-stick frying pan is ideal for this recipe.

3 medium eggs
1 tsp extra virgin olive oil
40g red onion, sliced
40g kale (weight with stalks removed), sliced
1 small garlic clove
½ tsp herbes de Provence
1 tsp chopped parsley,
20g cheese (feta, Cheddar, Lancashire or Wensleydale
    are our choices)

Heat the oven to 180°C/gas 4.

Crack the eggs into a bowl and whisk well.

Heat the olive oil in an ovenproof frying pan set over a low–medium heat and fry the onion, kale and garlic for 3–4 minutes or until soft.

Tip the cooked vegetables into the egg mix. Add the herbs and parsley and stir well. You can grate or crumble the cheese into the egg, depending on your preference.

Return the pan to a high heat and add the egg mixture. Leave on the heat for 30 seconds or until the egg starts to come away from the side of the pan. Transfer the pan to the oven.

Bake for 15 minutes, until the egg has set. If it is still a little runny in the centre, you can remove it from the oven and leave it to rest for 5 minutes before serving as the residual heat will continue to cook the frittata.

You could serve with a little rocket over the top and a drizzle of olive oil.

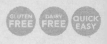

Lemon and herb sardines with rocket, avocado and caper salad

SERVES 1

juice of ½ lemon

30g red onion, sliced

30g celery, sliced

½ avocado

40g rocket

1 tsp capers

2 walnut halves, chopped

1 tsp extra virgin olive oil

120g drained tinned sardines (boneless are best, in olive oil or brine)

1 tbsp chopped parsley

Mix half the lemon juice with the red onion and celery. Slice the avocado and mix it with the rocket, capers, walnuts and olive oil.

Mix the sardines with the parsley and the rest of the lemon juice, then serve on top of the avocado and rocket mixture.

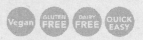

Bean and seaweed salad with miso dressing

SERVES 1

100g tinned or home-cooked mixed beans, drained and rinsed
5g arame or wakame, prepared as per the instructions on the packet
20g red onion, sliced
30g cucumber, diced
20g celery, sliced
40g rocket

For the miso dressing

1 tbsp miso paste
1 tsp extra virgin olive oil
1 tsp rice vinegar or white vinegar
juice of ½ lime
1 tsp chopped coriander
1 tsp sesame seeds

First make the dressing: whisk all the ingredients together and set to one side.

Mix all of the salad ingredients apart from the rocket in a bowl. Toss with the miso dressing and serve on a bed of the rocket.

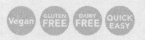

White bean, kale and sun-dried tomato salad

SERVES 1

30g kale (weight with stalks removed), finely sliced
1 tbsp pumpkin seeds
100g tinned or home-cooked beans, such as cannellini or
    haricot
25g sun-dried tomatoes, finely chopped
1 tsp chopped parsley
20g red onion, diced
20g celery, sliced
½ cooked beetroot, diced
10g pitted black olives
juice of ½ lemon
1 tsp extra virgin olive oil
40g rocket

Steam or boil the kale for around 5 minutes, until soft.
Drain and set aside.

Meanwhile, toast the pumpkin seeds in a dry frying pan,
then remove and set aside.

In a bowl mix the beans, tomatoes, parsley, onion, celery, beetroot and olives. Add the lemon juice and olive oil and mix well.

Stir the kale through the salad and serve on a bed of rocket, sprinkled with the pumpkin seeds.

MEAL 2

Chicken skewers with satay sauce and buckwheat

If you are using wooden skewers for this recipe, soak them in a little water for 10–15 minutes before using to prevent them burning while cooking.

150g chicken breast, cut into chunks
1 tsp ground turmeric
½ tsp extra virgin olive oil
50g buckwheat
30g kale (weight with stalks removed), sliced
30g celery, sliced
4 walnut halves, chopped, to garnish

For the sauce

20g red onion, diced
1 garlic clove, chopped
1 tsp extra virgin olive oil
1 tsp curry powder
1 tsp ground turmeric
50ml chicken stock
150ml coconut milk

117

1 tbsp walnut butter (shop-bought or see page 197), or
    peanut butter
1 tbsp chopped coriander

Mix the chicken with the turmeric and olive oil and set aside to marinate – 30 minutes to 1 hour would be best, but if you are short on time, just leave it for as long as you can.

Cook the buckwheat according to the packet instructions, adding the kale and celery for the last 5–7 minutes of the cooking time. Drain.

Heat the grill on a high setting.

For the sauce, gently fry the red onion and garlic in the olive oil for 2–3 minutes until soft. Add the spices and cook for a further minute. Add the stock and coconut milk and bring to the boil, then add the walnut butter and stir through. Reduce the heat and simmer the sauce for 8–10 minutes, or until creamy and rich.

As the sauce is simmering, thread the chicken on to the skewers and place under the hot grill for 10 minutes, turning them after 5 minutes.

To serve, stir the coriander through the sauce and pour it over the skewers, then scatter over the chopped walnuts.

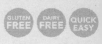

Baked cod with kale, chicory and white beans

SERVES 1

150g cod fillet
½ tsp extra virgin olive oil
1 tsp chopped parsley

For the beans

50g kale, sliced with the stalks removed
1 tsp extra virgin olive oil
30g red onion, sliced
1 garlic clove, chopped
100ml vegetable stock
75g tinned or home-cooked white beans, such as cannellini
   or haricot
1 head of chicory, halved lengthways and sliced

Heat the oven to 200°C/gas 6. Line a small baking tray with greaseproof paper.

Steam or boil the kale for 5–7 minutes until soft, then set aside.

Rub the fish in the olive oil and parsley, place on the prepared tray and bake in the oven for 10 minutes.

Meanwhile, heat the olive oil in a small saucepan over a low–medium heat and fry the red onion and garlic for 2–3 minutes, until soft. Add the stock and beans and bring to the boil. Add the chicory and cook for a further couple of minutes over a low–medium heat, taking care not to overcook it.

Stir the kale through the mixture and serve with the fish.

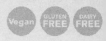

Tofu and chilli-baked chicory with rocket and walnut salad

SERVES 1

1 tsp extra virgin olive oil

30g red onion, diced

30g celery, diced

1 garlic clove, chopped

1 bird's eye chilli, chopped

1 tsp thyme (fresh or dried)

1 x 400g tin of tomatoes

150g silken tofu, cut into small cubes

1 tbsp chopped parsley

2 heads of chicory, quartered lengthways

For the salad

35g rocket

1 tsp capers

6 walnut halves, chopped

1 tsp extra virgin olive oil

1 tsp balsamic vinegar

Preheat the oven to 200°C/gas 6.

In a medium saucepan, heat the olive oil over a low–medium heat and cook the red onion, celery, garlic, chilli and thyme for 2–3 minutes or until soft.

Add the tomatoes and bring to the boil. Rinse the tin out with a little water and add the liquid to the pan. Leave to simmer for 10–15 minutes.

Add the tofu and parsley, taking care not to break up the tofu.

Lay the chicory in an ovenproof dish. Turn the oven up to 220°C/gas 7. Pour the hot sauce over the chicory and bake for 8–10 minutes, until the chicory is wilted and cooked.

Meanwhile, mix all the ingredients for the salad together in a bowl and serve with the chicory.

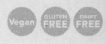

Asian marinated tofu with satay sauce and buckwheat with arame

If you are using wooden skewers for this recipe, soak them in a little water for 10–15 minutes before using to prevent them burning while cooking.

SERVES 1

150g firm tofu
½ tsp extra virgin olive oil
1 tsp tamari (or soy sauce if not avoiding gluten)
1 tsp ground turmeric
50g buckwheat
5g arame
2 walnut halves, chopped, to garnish (optional)

For the sauce

20g red onion, diced
1 garlic clove, chopped
1 tsp extra virgin olive oil
1 tsp ground turmeric
1 tsp curry powder

50ml vegetable stock

150ml coconut milk

1 tbsp walnut butter (shop-bought or see page 197), or
   peanut butter

1 tbsp chopped coriander

Drain the tofu and pat it dry with kitchen paper. Cut the tofu into bite-sized pieces and mix with the olive oil, tamari and turmeric. Set aside to marinate.

Cook the buckwheat and prepare the arame according to the instructions on their packets, then drain and mix them together.

Heat the grill on a high setting.

For the sauce, gently fry the red onion and garlic in the olive oil for 2–3 minutes until soft. Add the spices and cook for a further minute. Add the stock and coconut milk and bring to the boil, then add the walnut butter and stir through. Reduce the heat and simmer the sauce for 8–10 minutes or until creamy and rich, then stir through the coriander.

Thread the tofu pieces on to a skewer and grill for 8–10 minutes, turning once halfway through. They are ready when they are nicely browned.

Serve the tofu on a bed of buckwheat and drizzle the sauce over the top. Scatter over the chopped walnuts, if using.

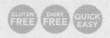

Quick tuna pasta

SERVES 1

75g buckwheat pasta
30g red onion, sliced
30g celery, sliced
30g kale (weight with stalks removed), finely sliced
1 garlic clove, chopped
1 tsp herbes de Provence
1 tsp extra virgin olive oil
100ml vegetable stock
1 tbsp chopped parsley
1 tsp capers
1 x 150g tin of tuna (in oil or brine), drained

Cook the pasta according to the packet instructions.

Meanwhile, cook the onion, celery, kale, garlic and dried
herbs in the olive oil over a low–medium heat for 3–4
minutes until they have softened.

Add the stock and cook for a further couple of minutes
on a similar heat. When all the vegetables are cooked to

your satisfaction, stir through the parsley, capers and tuna.

Add the cooked pasta, heat everything through and serve.

Thai stir-fried prawns or chicken with buckwheat

The paste for this recipe has a lot of ingredients but please don't be put off by that. If you have a food processor, it will do all the hard work for you, and if you can't find fresh lemongrass, you can omit it.

SERVES 1

50g buckwheat
1 tsp ground turmeric
125g chicken breast, sliced or cut into bite-sized pieces, **or**
    raw king prawns, peeled and deveined
40g celery, cut at an angle into 1cm slices
25g kale (weight with stalks removed), sliced
100ml chicken stock or vegetable stock
4–5 basil leaves

For the stir-fry paste

30g red onion, chopped
1 lemongrass stalk, bashed then chopped
1 garlic clove, chopped
1 bird's eye chilli, chopped

1 tsp ground turmeric

1 tsp ground cumin

1cm piece of fresh ginger, chopped

1 tsp extra virgin olive oil

1 tbsp chopped parsley

1 tsp fish sauce, soy sauce or tamari

Cook the buckwheat according to the instructions on the packet, with the turmeric stirred into the water.

Meanwhile, place all the paste ingredients in a food processor and blitz until you have a smooth paste. If you don't have a food processor, just chop everything as finely as possible and mix well.

Heat the paste in a frying pan over a medium heat. Add the chicken or prawns along with the celery and kale and cook for 4–5 minutes or until the chicken or prawns are cooked through. Add the stock and cook for a further 1–2 minutes.

Rip the basil leaves in half and add them to the pan. Serve with the buckwheat.

Grilled turkey escalope with a walnut, herb and Cheddar crust

If you can find only turkey steak, there are two ways to turn it into an escalope. Depending on how thick the steak is, you can either use a meat tenderiser, hammer or a rolling pin to bash it until it is around 5mm thick. Or, if you feel the steak is too thick for this to work, and you have a steady hand, cut the steak in half horizontally and then bash each piece with the tenderiser.

SERVES 1

150g turkey escalope or turkey breast steak
½ tsp extra virgin olive oil
10g Cheddar cheese, grated
1 tbsp chopped parsley
10g red onion, diced
10g walnuts, chopped
juice of ¼ lemon

For the salad

100g tomato wedges
40g rocket
20g red onions, sliced
1 tsp capers
30g celery, sliced
1 tsp extra virgin olive oil
1 tsp balsamic vinegar

Heat the grill on a high setting.

Rub the turkey with the olive oil, place on a baking sheet and grill for 4 minutes on each side.

Meanwhile, in a small bowl mix the cheese with the parsley, red onion and walnuts.

Toss all the ingredients for the salad together in a separate serving bowl.

When the turkey is cooked through, cover one side with the cheese mixture and return it to the grill for 2–3 minutes, or until the cheese and walnuts are starting to brown. Squeeze the lemon juice over the escalope and serve with the salad.

Lamb and date kofta with tzatziki, rocket and chilli buckwheat

There are four elements to this recipe but most of them are very simple and take no time at all.

SERVES 1

1 Medjool date, chopped
1 tsp ground turmeric
1 tsp ground cumin
20g red onion
1 tsp chopped parsley
1 medium egg yolk
1 small garlic clove
150g minced lamb

For the buckwheat

30g buckwheat
1 bird's eye chilli, chopped
1 tsp chopped parsley

For the tzatziki

50g natural yoghurt
20g cucumber, grated
½ tsp dried or fresh mint (optional)
juice of ¼ lemon

For the salad

50g tomato, diced
30g rocket
1 tsp extra virgin olive oil
juice of ¼ lemon

To make the kofta, place all the ingredients except the mince in a food processor and blitz until you have a smooth paste. Remove and knead this paste into the lamb. Shape the meat into two sausages and refrigerate for 30 minutes before cooking.

Cook the buckwheat according to the instructions on the packet.

For the tzatziki, simply mix all the ingredients together and set aside.

Heat the grill on a high setting.

Place your kofta under the grill for 8–10 minutes, turning them from time to time until they are nicely browned and cooked through.

Meanwhile, add the chopped chilli and parsley to the buckwheat and stir through.

For the salad, simply mix all the ingredients in a bowl.

Serve all the finished elements together.

Bunless beef burger with all the trimmings and sweet potato fries

SERVES 1

125g lean minced beef (5 per cent fat)
15g red onion, finely chopped
1 tsp finely chopped parsley
1 tsp extra virgin olive oil

For the fries

150g sweet potatoes
1 tsp extra virgin olive oil
1 tsp dried rosemary
1 garlic clove, unpeeled

To serve

10g Cheddar cheese, sliced or grated
150g red onion, sliced into rings
30g tomato, sliced
10g rocket
1 gherkin (optional)

Heat the oven to 220°C/gas 7.

Start by making the fries. Peel and cut the sweet potato into 1cm-thick chips. Toss them with the olive oil, rosemary and garlic clove. Place on a baking sheet and roast for 30 minutes, until nice and crispy.

For the burger, mix the onion and parsley with the minced beef. If you have pastry cutters, you could mould your burger with the largest pastry cutter in the set, otherwise, just use your hands to make a nice even patty.

Heat a frying pan over a medium heat, add the olive oil, then place the burger on one side of the pan and the onion rings on the other. Cook the burger for 6 minutes on each side, ensuring it is cooked through. Fry the onion rings until cooked to your liking.

When the burger is cooked, top it with the cheese and red onion and place it in the hot oven for a minute to melt the cheese. Remove and top with the tomato, rocket and gherkin. Serve with the fries.

Salmon tartare with rocket salad

We recommend using very fresh salmon then freezing it before preparing this dish. Leave the fish to defrost in the fridge overnight before use. A very sharp knife will be useful when you come to prepare it.

SERVES 1

125g skinless, boneless salmon fillet
20g red onion
1 tsp capers
1 tsp extra virgin olive oil
1 tbsp chopped parsley
juice of ¼ lemon
salt and pepper

For the salad

40g rocket
6 walnut halves, chopped
40g celery, sliced
1 tsp extra virgin olive oil
1 tsp balsamic vinegar

Cut the salmon fillet in half. Next cut each half into thin strips, then chop these into small dice.

Chop the red onion and capers as small as you can and mix them with the salmon. If you have a small food processor you could use this to chop them. Mix with the olive oil, parsley and a little salt and pepper.

Mix all the ingredients for the salad and serve with the salmon on top. Squeeze the lemon juice over the salmon and you're ready to go (do not add the lemon juice before serving as it will react with the raw fish and start to cook it).

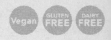

Stuffed portobello mushroom with braised celery

SERVES 1

50g tinned or home-cooked white beans, such as cannellini
  or haricot
1 tsp parsley
2 walnut halves
1 tbsp sunflower seeds
1 tsp extra virgin olive oil
30g red onion, sliced
20g kale (weight with stalks removed), sliced
1 garlic clove, chopped
1 large portobello mushroom
20g rocket, to serve

For the celery

3–4 celery sticks, cut in half
350ml vegetable stock
1 tsp dried thyme or 1 sprig of fresh thyme
1 garlic clove
1 tsp ground turmeric

Heat the oven to 180°C/gas 4.

For the celery, simply place all the ingredients in an ovenproof dish. Cover with a lid or foil and bake for 30–40 minutes, until tender.

While the celery is cooking, prepare your mushroom so that it's ready to go into the oven for the last 20 minutes or so of the celery cooking time. For the stuffing, blitz the beans, parsley and walnuts together in a food processor. If you don't have a food processor, simply mash the beans with the back of a fork and chop the parsley and walnuts as small as you can. Fold in the sunflower seeds.

Heat the olive oil in a small frying pan and gently cook the red onion, kale and garlic until soft. Remove from the heat and stir in the bean mixture. Stuff the mushroom with this, then place on a baking sheet.

Transfer to the oven and bake with the celery for the last 20–25 minutes of cooking time. The top of the mushroom should be nice and browned. Serve the mushrooms with the braised celery and rocket.

Arame and miso rissoles with crispy ginger kale

SERVES 1

5g arame
1 garlic clove, chopped
20g red onion, sliced
2 tsp extra virgin olive oil
75g tinned or home-cooked white beans, such as cannellini
   or haricot
150g silken tofu
20g miso paste
1 tbsp chopped coriander
2 tbsp sesame seeds

For the kale

1 tsp extra virgin olive oil
1cm piece of fresh ginger, chopped
80g kale (weight with stalks removed), chopped

Heat the oven to 180°C/gas 4.

First make the kale: rub the olive oil and ginger into it, place on a tray and bake for 25–30 minutes, turning it every 10 minutes to ensure it cooks evenly.

For the rissoles, prepare the arame according to the packet instructions. Gently fry the garlic and red onion in 1 teaspoon of the olive oil for 2–3 minutes. Pat the beans and tofu dry with kitchen paper, then place in a food processor with the miso and coriander. Blitz to a paste.

Drain and completely dry the arame before stirring it into the bean mixture. Shape into small patties and roll in the sesame seeds. Fry the rissoles in the remaining teaspoon of olive oil over a medium heat for 2–3 minutes on each side. They should turn a nice golden brown. Serve with the kale.

Maintenance

Welcome to Phase 2 of the Sirtfood Diet, or what we more aptly call 'Sirtfoods for life'. As good as the results of Phase 1 are, what really matters is being able to implement a Sirtfood-rich diet in the long term. That means making it part and parcel of everyday life. If you can achieve this, then the sky really is the limit as you continue to move towards your ideal weight. But remember, Sirtfoods are about so much more than just weight loss. By finding a sustainable and long-term way of eating, Sirtfoods are a culinary ticket to lifelong health and well-being. And, quite frankly, who's going to turn down the opportunity to feel amazing simply by eating delicious food?

So, what's the magic formula for success? It's actually very simple. Just eat the way you want to but with a big Sirtfood twist. It's not about counting the calories or the fats or the carbohydrates. Long-term success is only obtainable through focusing on what we gain through the food we put on our plates, not what you should be taking off. Sirtfoods for life offers the perfect way to achieve this; a way of eating where you know that every delicious mouthful does you good.

In broad terms, we recommend that you aim to base your daily diet around:

- 3 x Sirtfood-rich meals
- 1 x Sirtfood green juice or smoothie
- 1 x Sirtfood snack (optional)

To help you get that Sirtfood kickstart each day we recommend you continue with a daily Sirtfood green juice, best taken upon rising, before breakfast. To keep things interesting, we've included some variations of the classic Sirtfood green juice on pages 234–6.

Thereafter, it's a case of taking a balanced approach to breakfast, lunch and dinner, with the option of a Sirtfood-inspired snack if needed. Along with our popular Sirtfood bites, which we've included for you here for ease of reference (see page 190), we've provided a whole new bunch of snack ideas to keep you topped up on Sirtfood goodness.

We've worked hard to design recipes that fit into your lifestyle, not vice versa. So whether it's a grab-and-go breakfast, a packed lunch for the office, or a more decadent meal with friends (with dessert thrown into the bargain), we have you covered. True to form, family dinners are

covered too, and we've taken a fair share of everyday favourites and 'Sirtified' them. All you need to do is select recipes
from the relevant sections and you're up and running. It's
happy days as you get to eat the foods you love while
reaping all their benefits.

Of course if your diet were focused on just the top 20
Sirtfoods, no matter how good they are, things are going
to get monotonous sooner or later. Luckily, there are 40
foods that have moderate sirtuin-activating properties (see
pages 17–20 for the full list). We have liberally included
these in this part of the book, alongside the more familiar
top 20, to keep things varied and diverse, whilst still packing
a Sirtfood punch.

When all's said and done, the recipes that follow are
about establishing a way of eating that brings lifelong
health. What are you waiting for? Armed with your knife
and fork, it's time to tuck in.

BREAKFAST

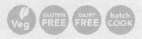

Sirt granola

Allow the granola to cool completely before storing it in an airtight container. Enjoy it with your choice of yoghurt and fresh strawberries, raspberries, blueberries, blackberries or chopped Medjool dates.

MAKES ABOUT 750G

50g coconut oil
150ml clear honey
1 tbsp ground turmeric
100g oats (use certified gluten-free oats if avoiding gluten)
250g buckwheat flakes
100g walnuts, chopped
50g pecans, chopped
50g flaked almonds
30g pumpkin seeds
30g sunflower seeds
50g cocoa nibs

Heat your oven to 160°C/gas 3.

In a small saucepan, melt the coconut oil and honey over a gentle heat, then stir in the turmeric. Mix well to ensure there are no lumps.

Mix all the dry ingredients together in a bowl and stir in the oil and honey. Make sure they are well combined, then transfer to a non-stick baking tray or one lined with baking paper. Bake for 35–40 minutes, stirring halfway through the cooking time.

Once it has achieved a nice golden colour, remove and leave to cool on the baking tray before storing in an airtight container for up to two months.

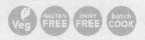

Sirt breakfast bars

The granola recipe on page 151 makes quite a large quantity, so if you get bored of granola on its own, you can make it into these delicious breakfast bites that can be eaten on the go or as a snack. All you will need is half the granola mixture.

MAKES ABOUT 10 BARS

150g pitted Medjool dates, chopped
150g walnut butter (shop-bought or see page 197)
50g thick honey
375g Sirtfood granola (see page 151)

Place the dates, walnut butter and honey in a food processor and blitz until you have a nice smooth paste. This may take some time as the dates will resist being pulped and you will have to scrape down the sides of the bowl a few times.

Transfer the paste to a mixing bowl and stir through the granola, making sure it is thoroughly combined. When you squeeze a lump of the mixture together in your hand it should remain solid.

Line a 25 x 18cm baking tin with greaseproof paper and spoon the mixture inside. Use your hands or the back of a spoon to spread it around the tin as evenly as possible, then pat it down firmly to ensure the bars stay in one piece when you slice them up. Alternatively, you could form the mixture into bite-sized balls.

Refrigerate for at least 2 hours before attempting to cut the mixture into about 10 bars. You can then store them in an airtight container in the fridge for up to two weeks.

Sirt 'cocoa pops'

This recipe can be made vegan and dairy-free if you use a dairy-free milk such as almond or soya.

MAKES ABOUT 10 SERVINGS

100g popping corn
1 tbsp extra virgin olive oil or melted coconut oil

For the topping

50g walnuts, chopped
50g sunflower seeds
50g buckwheat flakes
35g cocoa nibs

To serve

1 tsp cocoa powder (100 per cent)
1 Medjool date, finely chopped
200ml milk or dairy-free alternative

Heat the oven to 160°C/gas 3.

Place a heavy-based pan with a tight-fitting lid over a medium heat. Mix the corn and oil together, then add the mixture to the hot pan and cover with the lid. Shake the pan to keep the corn moving inside it. As soon as it starts to pop, turn up the heat and keep shaking the pan as much as you can with the lid still on. Once the popping calms down to around 2–3 seconds between each pop, remove the pan from the heat and empty it into a bowl. Discard any unpopped kernels, allow to cool completely, then transfer to an airtight container and store for up to a week.

For the topping, place the walnuts and sunflower seeds in a small baking tray and toast in the oven for 15 minutes. Transfer to a bowl and mix with the buckwheat and cocoa nibs. Allow to cool completely, then store in an airtight container for up to 1 month.

The popped corn and topping should be stored separately to ensure an even distribution when serving.

To serve, measure 1–2 tablespoons of the topping and 10g of the popcorn into a bowl. Stir the cocoa powder and date into the milk, then pour it over the cereal.

Sirt fruit bowl

SERVES 1

40g (10) raspberries
60g (10) red/black grapes, halved
80g (1 medium) stoned plum, chopped
60g (½ medium) apple, sliced
50g (2 medium) hulled strawberries, chopped
juice of ¼ lemon
100g Greek yoghurt
5 walnut halves, crushed

Put all the fruit together in a bowl. Squeeze the lemon juice over it and mix well.

Pour over the Greek yoghurt, scatter the crushed walnuts on top and serve.

Grilled sausages with fried onions and herb scrambled eggs

SERVES 1

2 lean pork or beef sausages
2 eggs
1 tsp chopped parsley
1 tsp chopped chives
25ml milk or dairy-free alternative
1 tsp extra virgin olive oil
60g red onion
1 tsp dried thyme

Heat a grill on its highest setting.

Grill the sausages for 8–10 minutes, turning them from time to time until they are nicely browned all over.

Whisk the eggs, parsley, chives and milk together. Add ½ teaspoon of the olive oil to a small saucepan placed over a medium heat, add the egg mixture and cook gently until you have a nice scramble.

Meanwhile, put the remaining ½ teaspoon of olive oil in a small frying pan over a medium heat and fry the onion and thyme for 3–4 minutes until they are browned.

Pile the eggs on to a plate and top with the sausages and onion.

Smoked salmon, rocket and capers on buckwheat crackers

SERVES 1

1 tsp capers
60g Greek yoghurt
1 tbsp chopped parsley
10g red onion, thinly sliced
buckwheat crackers (shop-bought or home-made: see page
   193 to make your own)
75g smoked salmon
20g rocket
juice of ¼ lemon

Mix the capers, yoghurt, parsley and onion together in a bowl. Divide the mixture between your crackers, then top with the smoked salmon and rocket. Squeeze over some lemon juice to finish.

Baked kippers with kale and poached eggs

Kippers have been a much maligned food over recent years. Yes, they do have a very distinctive smell, but the sweet and smoky flavour is something worth bringing into your life. We've chosen to bake our kippers but you could easily poach or grill yours. Some supermarkets sell them as 'boil in the bag', which are also fine. You will need to time things carefully so that the different elements are ready together.

1 kipper
1 tsp extra virgin olive oil
1 tsp chopped parsley
50g kale, chopped
a few drops of vinegar
1 medium egg
1 lemon wedge

Heat your oven to 200°C/gas 6. Meanwhile, bring 2 small saucepans of water to the boil.

Cut the head and tail off your kipper, if necessary, and place skin-side down on a piece of foil. Spoon the olive oil and parsley over the kipper and wrap the foil around it.

Place the kale in one pan of boiling water and simmer for 5 minutes, or until tender. Drain and keep warm.

Add a few drops of vinegar to the other pan of boiling water and reduce the heat to a simmer. Stir the water in a clockwise motion, then crack your egg into the centre of the whirlpool. An egg with a firm white and runny yolk will take 2–3 minutes, depending on its freshness. Remove with a slotted spoon and drain on kitchen paper.

Serve the egg on top of the kipper with the kale to the side, or however you prefer.

Poached egg with rocket, asparagus and bacon

SERVES 1

2 slices of streaky or back bacon
6 asparagus spears, woody ends snapped off
a few drops of vinegar
2 eggs
10g rocket
1 tsp extra virgin olive oil

Heat a grill on its highest setting. Meanwhile, bring 2 small saucepans of water to the boil.

Once the grill is hot, grill your bacon until the fat has started to crisp – it should take 4–5 minutes.

Place the asparagus spears in one pan of boiling water and cook for 2–3 minutes until softened.

Add a few drops of vinegar to the other pan of boiling water and reduce the heat to a simmer. Stir the water in a clockwise motion, then crack an egg into the centre of the whirlpool. An egg with a firm white and runny yolk will take 2–3 minutes, depending on its freshness. Remove with a slotted spoon and drain on kitchen paper. Cook the second egg in the same way.

Serve the eggs on top of the asparagus, top with the crispy bacon and rocket, then drizzle over the olive oil.

LUNCH

Sirt smoked mackerel pâté with celery sticks

You could serve this pâté with a watercress and caper salad and some buckwheat crackers (see page 193) instead of the celery if you prefer.

SERVES 1

1 smoked mackerel fillet (80–90g), skinned
1 tbsp chopped parsley
1 tsp extra virgin olive oil
1 tbsp crème fraîche
1 tbsp cream cheese
pinch of cayenne pepper
freshly ground black pepper
juice of ¼–½ lemon, according to taste
2–3 sticks of celery, depending on size

Place three-quarters of the fish in a food processor. Add the remaining ingredients, except the celery, and blitz until you have a smooth paste.

Transfer to a bowl and flake the remaining fish into the pâté to give it some texture.

Cut the celery into 5cm lengths and serve with the pâté.

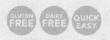

Tuna niçoise salad

SERVES 1

50g green beans
1 medium egg
20g celery, diced
50g cherry tomatoes, cut in half
20g red onion, thinly sliced
15g small black olives
1 tsp chopped parsley
2 tsp extra virgin olive oil
½ tsp white wine vinegar
20g rocket
1 x 150g tin of tuna (in oil or brine), drained
juice of ¼–½ lemon, according to taste

Bring a small saucepan of water to the boil. Once boiling, cook the beans for 3-6 minutes depending on how crunchy you like them, then remove with a slotted spoon and set aside.

Boil the egg in the same water. If straight from the fridge, we find simmering the egg for 7 minutes leaves you with a firm white and slightly runny yolk. Cook for a full 10 minutes if you prefer a solid yolk. Once the time is up, place the egg under running cold water until cool enough to handle, then peel and set aside.

Mix the celery, tomatoes, onion, olives, beans and parsley together with the olive oil and vinegar.

Place this salad on top the rocket. Cut the egg into quarters and add them, then flake the tuna meat around the plate. Squeeze some lemon juice over the tuna to finish.

Buckwheat pasta salad with artichoke, Parmesan and Parma ham

SERVES 1

60g buckwheat pasta
50g tinned artichokes (in oil or water), drained and cut into
    bite-sized pieces
130g (1) tomato, diced or cut into 8 wedges
1 tsp capers
10g red onion, thinly sliced
1 tsp extra virgin olive oil
juice of ¼–½ lemon, according to taste
1 tbsp chopped parsley
2 slices of Parma ham or other cured ham
20g rocket
15g Parmesan or other hard Italian cheese

Cook the pasta according to the instructions on the packet, then drain well and set aside.

In a bowl mix the artichokes, tomato, capers, red onion, olive oil, lemon juice and parsley. Toss with the cooked pasta.

Slice or rip the ham into 3–4 pieces and mix through the pasta. Place the pasta on top of the rocket, grate or shave the Parmesan over the top and serve.

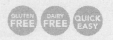

Chicken, quinoa and avocado salad

SERVES 1

50g quinoa
20g red onion, thinly sliced
1 tsp capers
1 tbsp chopped parsley
20g sun-dried tomatoes finely chopped
1 tsp extra virgin olive oil
juice of ¼–½ lemon, according to taste
100g cooked chicken breast, cut into bite-sized pieces
½ avocado, sliced
20g rocket

Cook the quinoa as directed on the packet, then drain well and transfer to a bowl.

Mix the onion, capers, parsley, sun-dried tomatoes, olive oil and lemon juice together, then stir this mixture through the cooked quinoa.

Add the chicken and avocado to the quinoa mix and serve on top of the rocket.

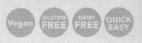

15-minute watercress soup

For a more substantial lunch, serve the soup with our buckwheat and seed crackers (see page 193).

SERVES 1

2 tsp extra virgin olive oil
30g celery, thinly sliced
30g white onion, thinly sliced
200ml vegetable stock
50g tinned or home-cooked white beans such as cannellini or haricot
75g watercress
1 tbsp chopped parsley

Place 1 teaspoon of the olive oil in a small saucepan and gently cook the celery and onion for 2 minutes. Add the stock and beans, bring to the boil and cook over a medium heat for 10 minutes.

Roughly chop the watercress and parsley, add them to the pan and cook for 1 minute. Remove from the heat and blend until smooth.

Serve the soup drizzled with the remaining teaspoon of olive oil.

Broccoli, blue cheese and basil soup

For a more substantial lunch, serve the soup with our buckwheat and seed crackers (see page 193).

SERVES 1

2 tsp extra virgin olive oil

30g red onion, sliced

30g celery, sliced

125g broccoli (including the stalks), sliced

1 small garlic clove, sliced

½ tsp dried thyme

50g tinned or home-cooked white beans such as cannellini or haricot

500ml vegetable stock

20g blue cheese

4–5 basil leaves

Place 1 teaspoon of the olive oil in a saucepan and fry the onion, celery, broccoli, garlic and thyme over a low–medium heat for 2–3 minutes.

Add the beans and stock and bring to the boil. Cook for 30 minutes over a low heat until all the vegetables are soft.

Add the blue cheese and blend until smooth. Rip the basil leaves apart and add to the finished soup. Serve drizzled with the remaining teaspoon of olive oil.

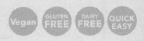

Edamame and noodle salad

SERVES 1

65g buckwheat noodles
30g red onion, thinly sliced
1 bird's eye chilli, thinly sliced
30g celery, thinly sliced
30g carrot, grated
75g shelled edamame beans

For the dressing

1–2cm piece of fresh ginger
juice of ¼ lime
1 tsp tamari (or soy sauce if not avoiding gluten)
2 tsp extra virgin olive oil
1 tbsp chopped coriander
1 tsp sesame seeds

Cook the noodles according to the instructions on the packet. Drain in a colander, rinse with cold water, and leave them to cool.

To make the dressing grate the ginger into a bowl and add the lime juice, tamari, olive oil, coriander and sesame seeds.

Combine the red onion, chilli, celery, carrot and beans in a bowl. Add the noodles and dressing, toss well and serve.

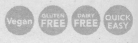

Broccoli, bean and artichoke salad

SERVES 1

60g broccoli florets

75g tinned or home-cooked white beans such as cannellini or
  haricot

20g red onion, thinly sliced

40g tinned artichokes (in oil or brine), cut into quarters

15g small black olives

1 tbsp chopped parsley

juice of ¼–½ lemon, according to taste

1 tsp extra virgin olive oil

30g rocket

1 tbsp pumpkin seeds, toasted

Finely chop the broccoli until it roughly resembles the
texture of couscous. Alternatively, you could place the
broccoli in a food processor to achieve a similar result –
use the pulse setting to avoid overworking it.

Mix all the remaining ingredients, except the rocket and
pumpkin seeds, in a bowl.

Place the broccoli mixture on top of the rocket, scatter over the pumpkin seeds and serve.

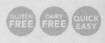

Smoked trout, watercress and new potato salad

This is best served while the potatoes are still warm so that they absorb the dressing.

You could swap the smoked trout for smoked salmon if you wish.

SERVES 1

100g new potatoes
1 tsp capers
1 tsp extra virgin olive oil
1 tsp chopped parsley
20g red onion, thinly sliced
20g celery, thinly sliced
juice of ¼–½ lemon, according to taste
100g smoked trout
35g watercress, roughly chopped

Depending on the size of your potatoes, either cut them in half or cook them whole in a pan of simmering water for 15–20 minutes.

In a bowl mix the capers, olive oil, parsley, red onion, celery and lemon juice.

Drain the potatoes and using the back of a fork give them a little press to open them up a little. You don't want to mash them, so be gentle. While they are still warm, combine them with the caper mixture.

Tear or slice the smoked trout and mix it with the watercress. Serve immediately over the cooked potatoes. You could squeeze some more lemon juice over to finish if you like.

Sirt green bean salad

SERVES 1

20g red onion, thinly sliced

1 tsp red wine vinegar (or white or cider vinegar)

150g green beans, topped and tailed

50g tinned or home-cooked white beans such as cannellini or
haricot

4–6 walnut halves, chopped

1 tsp capers

100g tomato, diced

2 tsp extra virgin olive oil

1 tsp chopped chives

1 tsp chopped parsley

25g rocket

25g feta cheese

squeeze of lemon juice (optional)

Place the sliced onion in the vinegar and set aside to
marinate. This will soften and sweeten the onion.

Cook the green beans in boiling water for 4–6 minutes depending on how crunchy you like them. Drain in a colander and run cold water over them until cool.

Combine the beans, walnuts, capers, tomato, oil, and herbs in a bowl, then stir in the vinegar and onion mixture. Serve on top of the rocket and crumble over the feta cheese. Finish it with a squeeze of lemon juice if you wish.

DRESSINGS

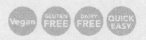

Rocket and caper salad dressing

To help you Sirtify any salad, we've put together two easy dressings to have at hand in the fridge.

MAKES ABOUT 250ML

200ml extra virgin olive oil
30ml white wine vinegar
20ml lemon juice
1 tsp capers
1 tsp chopped parsley
5g chopped rocket

Place all the ingredients in a jug and blend with a stick blender for a minute or so. Once emulsified into a smooth dressing, place in a screwtop jar or airtight container and store in the fridge – the dressing will keep for up to a week.

If you find that the dressing separates, simply give it a shake before using. You might also find that you need to remove it from the fridge 10–15 minutes before using as it may set a little.

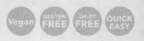

Chilli and turmeric salad dressing

MAKES ABOUT 250ML

200ml extra virgin olive oil
30ml white wine vinegar
20ml lemon juice
1 bird's eye chilli, chopped
1 tsp ground turmeric
½ tsp English or Dijon mustard

Place all the ingredients in a jug and blend with a stick
blender for a minute or so. Once emulsified into a
smooth dressing, place in a screwtop jar or airtight
container and store in the fridge – the dressing will keep
for up to a week.

If the dressing separates, simply give it a shake before
using. You might also find that you need to remove it
from the fridge 10–15 minutes before using as it may set
a little.

SNACKS

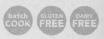

Sirtfood bites

MAKES 15–20

120g walnuts
30g dark chocolate (85 per cent cocoa solids), broken into
    pieces, or cocoa nibs
250g Medjool dates, pitted
1 tbsp cocoa powder (100 per cent)
1 tbsp ground turmeric
1 tbsp extra virgin olive oil
seeds from 1 vanilla pod or 1 tsp vanilla extract
1–2 tbsp water (optional)

Place the walnuts and chocolate in a food processor
and blitz until you have a fine powder. Add all the
other ingredients except the water and blend until the
mixture forms a ball. You can add the water if the
mixture seems dry, but take care – you don't want it to
be too sticky.

Using your hands, form the mixture into bite-sized balls
and refrigerate in an airtight container for at least 1 hour
before eating them. To achieve a different finish, roll

some of the balls in more cocoa powder, or desiccated coconut if you like. The bites will keep for up to 1 week in the fridge.

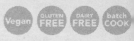

Toasted Cajun nuts

MAKES 250G

250g blanched peanuts or a mix of pecans, walnuts and
   hazelnuts
1 tbsp extra virgin olive oil or coconut oil
1 tsp paprika
1 tsp dried thyme
1 tsp sea salt
1 tsp oregano
1 tsp chilli powder

Heat the oven to 160°C/gas 3.

Mix all the spices together and combine with the nuts
and oil. Place the nuts in a single layer in roasting tray
and roast for 25–30 minutes. (You might have to cook
them in batches.) Tip the toasted nuts into a bowl.

When completely cool, store in an airtight container for
up to two days.

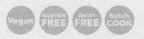

Buckwheat and seed crackers

MAKES ABOUT 40

200g buckwheat flour
50g sunflower seeds
50g pumpkin seeds
35g sesame seeds
1 tbsp extra virgin olive oil
150ml water

Place all the ingredients in a mixing bowl and combine them thoroughly using your hands. Leave to sit for 30 minutes, covered with a tea towel or some cling film. The mix may seem a bit wet to begin with but the water will be absorbed while the dough rests.

Heat the oven to 160°C/gas 3. Line a large baking tray with non-stick baking paper.

Remove the dough from the bowl and use your hands to work it into a nice ball. You might have to add a little water if it feels a bit dry.

Divide the dough in half, place on a lightly floured work surface roll it out to a thickness of about 1–2mm. You can either bake the dough as single pieces and then break them up, or cut them into 5–7cm rounds. Re-roll any off-cuts and stamp out more circles until you have used all the dough. Repeat with the other half of the dough – in total you should have around 40 crackers. Transfer the dough to the lined tray (you might need to bake them in two batches, depending on the size of your tray).

Bake for 15–20 minutes, until lightly brown and firm to the touch. The timing depends on how crunchy you like the finished product. The crackers can be kept in an airtight container for up to 7 days.

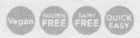

Sea salt and cider vinegar popcorn

SERVES 2

50g popping corn
1 tbsp extra virgin olive oil
1 tbsp apple cider vinegar
1 tsp sea salt

Place a heavy-based saucepan with a tight-fitting lid over a medium heat. Mix the corn and oil together, then add the mixture to the hot pan and cover with the lid. Shake the pan to keep the corn moving inside it. As soon as it starts to pop, turn up the heat and keep shaking the pan as much as you can with the lid still on. Once the popping calms down to around 2–3 seconds between each pop, remove the pan from the heat and empty it into a bowl. Discard any unpopped kernels.

Shake the salt and vinegar over the popcorn and serve while warm.

The popcorn will keep for up to a week in an airtight container.

Other tasty seasonings you could try

hot smoked paprika
curry powder
olive oil and dried oregano
cocoa powder
grated Parmesan

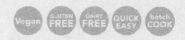

Walnut butter

MAKES 350G

350g walnuts
2 tsp extra virgin olive oil
1 tsp water

Simply place the walnuts in a food processor and blitz
for around 2 minutes until you have fine crumbs.
Gradually add the oil and water and continue until you
have a smooth butter.

This can be kept for up to 1 week if stored in an airtight
container in your fridge.

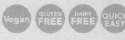

Sirt ants on a log

A fun children's snack gets Sirtified.

SERVES 1

3 celery sticks
60g walnut butter (see page 197)
3 Medjool dates, chopped

Cut each celery stick into three lengths. Using a knife, spread the walnut butter along the central hollow of each piece and top with the dates.

DINNER

Beef bourguignon with mashed potatoes and kale

SERVES 4

800g diced stewing beef (chuck or shin)

2–3 tbsp buckwheat flour

1 tbsp extra virgin olive oil

150g red onion, roughly chopped

200g celery, roughly chopped

100g carrot, roughly chopped

2–3 garlic cloves, chopped

375ml red wine

2 tbsp tomato purée

750ml beef stock

2 bay leaves

1 sprig of fresh thyme or 1 tbsp dried thyme

75g diced pancetta or smoked lardons

250g button mushrooms

2 tbsp chopped parsley

200g kale

1 tbsp cornflour or arrowroot (optional)

For the mash

500g Maris Piper or King Edward potatoes
1 tbsp extra virgin olive oil
1 tbsp milk

Pat the beef dry with kitchen paper if there is a lot of blood, then roll it in the flour. Heat a heavy-based saucepan over a medium–high heat. Add the olive oil, then the beef and cook the meat until it is nicely browned all over. It is best to do this in 3–4 small batches, depending on the size of your pan. When all the meat is brown, remove from the pan using a slotted spoon and set aside.

To the same pan add the onion, celery, carrot and garlic and sweat for 3–4 minutes over a medium heat, until softened. Add the wine, tomato purée and stock and bring to the boil. Add the browned beef, bay leaves and thyme and reduce the heat to a simmer. Cover the pan with a lid and cook for 2 hours, stirring from time to time to make sure nothing sticks to the bottom.

While the beef is cooking, peel your potatoes and cut them into quarters (or smaller chunks if they are quite large). Place in a pan of cold water and bring to the boil. Reduce the heat to a simmer and cook for 20–25 minutes, covered with a lid. When soft, drain and mash with the olive oil and milk. Keep warm.

While the potatoes are cooking, heat a frying pan over a high heat. When hot but not smoking, add the diced pancetta. The fat content of the bacon means you won't need any oil to cook it. When some of the fat has been released and it is starting to brown, add the mushrooms and cook over a medium heat until both are nicely browned. You might have to do this in a couple of batches, depending on the size of your pan. When cooked, place to one side.

Boil or steam the kale for 5–10 minutes, until tender.

Once the beef is tender enough and the sauce thickened to your liking, add the pancetta, mushrooms and parsley. If your sauce is still a little runny you could mix the cornflour or arrowroot with a little water, then stir the paste into the sauce until you have your desired consistency. Cook for 2–3 minutes and serve with the mash and kale.

Turkey fajitas

This Mexican favourite is just as good with chicken or king prawns.

SERVES 4

For the filling

500g turkey breast meat, cut into strips
1 tbsp extra virgin olive oil
1–2 bird's eye chillies, according to taste, chopped
150g red onion, thinly sliced
150g red pepper, cut into thin strips
2–3 garlic cloves, chopped
1 tbsp paprika
1 tbsp ground cumin
1 tsp chilli powder
1 tbsp chopped coriander

For the guacamole

2 ripe avocados, peeled and stoned (reserve one of the
    stones)
juice of 1 lime

pinch of chilli powder
pinch of black pepper

For the salsa

1 x 400g tin of chopped tomatoes
20g red onion, diced
20g red pepper, deseeded and diced
juice of ½–1 lime, depending on size
1 tsp chopped coriander
1 tsp capers

For the salad

100g rocket
3 tomatoes, sliced
100g cucumber, thinly sliced
1 tbsp extra virgin olive oil
juice of ½ lemon

To serve

100g Cheddar cheese, grated
8 wholemeal tortilla wraps

Mix the filling ingredients together, then set aside while
you prepare the other parts.

Place all the guacamole ingredients in a small food processor and blitz until you have a smooth paste. Alternatively, you can mash them all together with the back of a fork or spoon. Place the reserved avocado stone in the guacamole – it will stop it from going brown.

Mix all the ingredients for the salsa. If you would like extra heat add some chopped bird's eye chilli.

Toss all the salad ingredients in a large bowl.

Place your largest frying pan over a high heat until it starts to smoke. Have the overhead fan on if you have one as this will create smoke. Add the turkey filling to the hot pan – you might need to cook it in 2–3 batches because overloading the pan creates too much moisture and it will start boiling instead of frying. Keep the pan over a high heat and keep moving the mix around so that the turkey colours nicely but doesn't burn. Keep the cooked meat warm in a low oven.

To serve, reheat the tortillas according to the packet instructions, then spread some guacamole over each wrap; top with some cheese, a little salsa and then pile the turkey mix in the middle and roll it up like a big cigar. Serve the salad alongside.

Sirt chicken korma

If you prefer, you could replace the chicken thighs with breast fillets, cut them into 6–8 pieces and reduce the cooking time to 20 minutes. If you like your curry to have more of a kick, simply add 1–2 bird's eye chillies to the paste.

SERVES 4

350ml chicken stock
30g Medjool date, chopped
2 cinnamon sticks
4–5 cardamom pods, slightly split
250ml coconut milk
8 boneless, skinless chicken thighs
1 tbsp ground turmeric
200g buckwheat
150ml Greek yoghurt
50g ground walnuts
2 tbsp chopped coriander

For the curry paste

1 large red onion, quartered
3 garlic cloves

2cm piece of fresh ginger

1 tbsp mild curry powder

1 tsp ground cumin

1 tbsp ground turmeric

1 tbsp coconut oil

Place the ingredients for the curry paste in a food processor and blitz for around a minute until you have a nice paste. You will have to scrape the sides down from time to time to achieve this. Alternatively you could grind it using a pestle and mortar.

Cook the paste in a heavy-based pan over a medium heat for 1–2 minutes, then add the stock, date, cinnamon, cardamom pods and coconut milk. Bring to the boil, then add the chicken thighs. Reduce the heat, cover the pan with a lid and leave to simmer for 45 minutes.

Meanwhile, bring a pan of water to the boil and stir in the turmeric. Add the buckwheat and cook according to the instructions on the packet.

Once the chicken is tender, stir in the yoghurt and walnuts cook for a further couple of minutes over a low heat. Add the coriander and serve with the buckwheat.

Prawn, pak choi and broccoli stir-fry

SERVES 4

1 tbsp ground turmeric
400g raw prawns, shelled and deveined
1 tbsp coconut oil
280g buckwheat noodles
1 tsp extra virgin olive oil

For the stir-fry

1 tbsp coconut oil
250g broccoli, cut into bite-sized pieces
250g pak choi, roughly chopped
1 red onion, thinly sliced
2cm piece of fresh ginger, chopped
1–2 bird's eye chillies, chopped
3 garlic cloves, chopped
150ml vegetable stock
1 bunch of basil, leaves removed and stalks chopped
1 tbsp Thai fish sauce or tamari

Mix the turmeric with the prawns. Place the coconut oil in a wok or frying pan and cook the prawns over a medium–high heat for 3–4 minutes or until they're opaque. Once cooked, remove from the pan and set aside.

For the stir-fry, wipe out the pan and place it over a high heat until it starts to smoke. Add the coconut oil, then add the vegetables, ginger, chillies and garlic. Keep moving the vegetables around the pan so they don't burn. Cook for 3–5 minutes – lower the heat a little if the vegetables look like they're charring – until cooked but crunchy. Add the stock, all the basil and fish sauce. Bring to the boil, then add the prawns, letting heat them through.

Meanwhile, cook the noodles according to the instructions on the packet. Refresh in cold water and mix with the olive oil to stop them sticking together.

Serve the stir-fry with the hot noodles.

Cocoa spaghetti bolognese

SERVES 4

1 tbsp extra virgin olive oil

1 red onion, finely diced

100g celery, finely diced

100g carrot, finely diced

3 garlic cloves, chopped

400g lean minced beef (5 per cent fat)

1 tbsp herbes de Provence

1–2 bay leaves

150ml red wine

300ml beef stock

1 tbsp cocoa powder (100 per cent)

1 tbsp tomato purée

2 x 400g tins of chopped tomatoes

280g wholemeal spaghetti

1 tsp ground black pepper

1 bunch of fresh basil, leaves only

20g Parmesan cheese

Heat the oil in a pan, then cook the onion, celery, carrot and garlic over a medium heat for 1–2 minutes, until softened a little.

Add the mince and dried herbs and cook over a medium–high heat until the mince is browned. Add the wine, stock, cocoa powder, tomato purée and tinned tomatoes, bring to the boil and leave to simmer for 45–60 minutes with a lid on.

When almost ready to serve, cook the pasta as directed on the packet.

To finish, stir the pepper and basil leaves into the sauce. Serve with the pasta and grate some Parmesan over the top.

Baked salmon with watercress sauce and new potatoes

SERVES 4

400g new potatoes
4 x 125g skinless salmon fillets
1 tsp extra virgin olive oil
1 head of broccoli, cut into florets
1 bunch of asparagus spears, woody ends snapped off

For the watercress sauce

30g watercress
5g parsley
1 tbsp capers
2 tbsp extra virgin olive oil
juice of 1 lemon

Heat the oven to 200°C/gas 6.

Place the potatoes in a pan of cold water. Bring to the boil and simmer for 15–20 minutes or until tender.

Brush the salmon fillets with the olive oil, place on a baking tray and bake in the oven for 10 minutes. Reduce the cooking time by 2–3 minutes if you prefer your salmon lightly cooked.

Meanwhile, boil or steam the broccoli and asparagus until tender.

Put the ingredients for the sauce in a food processor or blender and blitz until smooth.

Serve the salmon with the sauce poured over and the vegetables alongside.

Coq au vin with new potatoes and green beans

SERVES 4

4 skinless chicken thighs

4 skinless chicken drumsticks

1–2 tbsp buckwheat flour

1 tbsp extra virgin olive oil

150g red onion

150g carrot

200g celery

3 garlic cloves, chopped

400ml red wine

400ml chicken stock

1 sprig of fresh thyme

2–3 bay leaves

100g pancetta or smoked bacon, diced

250g button mushrooms

400g new potatoes

2 tbsp chopped parsley

250g green beans, topped and tailed

Roll the chicken pieces in the flour. Heat a heavy-based saucepan over a medium–high heat. Add the olive oil, then the chicken and cook until it is nicely browned all over. Remove from the pan and set aside.

To the same pan add the onion, carrot, celery and garlic and cook gently for 2–3 minutes until they have started to soften. You could add a little splash of water here if the pan has gone dry. Add the wine and chicken stock and bring to the boil. Add the thyme, bay leaves and chicken. Cover with a lid and simmer gently for 45 minutes checking the amount of liquid from time to time and adding a little more.

Heat a frying pan over a high heat. When hot but not smoking, add the diced pancetta. When some of the fat has been released and it is starting to brown, add the mushrooms and cook over a medium heat until both they and the pancetta are nicely browned. You might have to do this in a couple of batches, depending on the size of your pan. When cooked, place to one side.

Place the potatoes in a pan of cold water. Bring to the boil and simmer for 15–20 minutes or until tender. When ready, drain and return to the pan to keep warm.

Add the pancetta, mushrooms and parsley to the coq au vin and cook for a further 15 minutes.

To cook the green beans either steam or boil them for 4–6 minutes, depending on how crunchy you like them. Serve the coq au vin with the potatoes and beans alongside.

Salmon and buckwheat pasta bake

This can be served with some steamed broccoli
or a simple rocket salad.

SERVES 4

300g skinless salmon fillet
1 tsp extra virgin olive oil
250g buckwheat pasta
100g kale, chopped
1 large courgette, cut lengthways into quarters and sliced
1 red onion, sliced
4 garlic cloves, chopped
1 tbsp herbes de Provence
1 tbsp extra virgin olive oil

For the sauce

650ml milk or dairy-free alternative
65g unsalted butter
65g buckwheat or plain flour
150g Cheddar cheese, grated

2 tbsp chopped parsley
2 tbsp capers

Heat the oven to 200°C/gas 6.

Rub the salmon with the olive oil and place it on a piece of foil. Fold over and seal the edges to make a parcel. Bake in the oven for 15 minutes.

Cook the pasta according to the instructions on the packet. Drain, then pour over some warm water from the kettle to stop it sticking, and place to one side.

To make the sauce, bring the milk to the boil in a small saucepan, taking care that it doesn't spill over. Next melt the butter in a separate pan and add the flour. Mix together until you have a mixture that is neither too wet nor too dry. You may have to add a little more flour or butter to achieve this. On a low heat gently cook this for 30 seconds to 1 minute until it leaves the side of the pan. Gradually add the hot milk, stirring continuously until you have a nice thick sauce. Add 100g of the cheese, the parsley and capers and remove from the heat.

Meanwhile, boil or steam the kale until tender.

In a frying pan set over a medium heat, cook the courgette, red onion, garlic and herbs in the olive oil for 2–3 minutes until softened. Mix with the cooked kale.

Heat a grill on its highest setting.

Flake the cooked salmon and mix with the pasta, cooked vegetables and sauce, transfer to an ovenproof dish and scatter over the remaining cheese. Place under the hot grill for 5 minutes, until the cheese starts to brown.

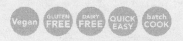

Cauliflower and kale curry

SERVES 4

200g buckwheat
2 tbsp ground turmeric
1 red onion, chopped
3 garlic cloves, chopped
2.5cm piece of fresh ginger, chopped
1–2 bird's eye chillies, chopped
1 tbsp coconut oil
1 tbsp mild curry powder
1 tbsp ground cumin
2 x 400g tins of chopped tomatoes
300ml vegetable stock
200g kale, roughly sliced
300g cauliflower, chopped
1 x 400g tin of butter beans, drained and rinsed
2 tomatoes, cut into wedges
2 tbsp chopped coriander

Cook the buckwheat according to the instructions on the packet, adding 1 tablespoon of the turmeric to the water.

Meanwhile, cook the onion, garlic, ginger and chillies in the coconut oil for 2–3 minutes over a medium heat. Add the spices, including the remaining tablespoon of turmeric, and continue to cook over a low–medium heat for 1–2 minutes.

Add the tinned tomatoes and stock and bring to the boil, then simmer for 10 minutes. Add the kale, cauliflower and butter beans and cook for 10 minutes. Add the tomato wedges and coriander and cook for a further minute, then serve with the buckwheat.

Kidney bean burritos

SERVES 4

1 tbsp extra virgin olive oil

1 red onion, diced

3 garlic cloves, chopped

1 bird's eye chilli, chopped

1 tbsp paprika

1 tbsp ground cumin

1 tsp chilli powder

1 tbsp chopped coriander

2 tomatoes, chopped

3 x 400g tins of kidney beans, drained and rinsed

500ml vegetable stock

150g Cheddar or vegan cheese

8 wholemeal tortilla wraps

1 x 500g jar of tomato passata

1 x 200g jar of jalepeño peppers (optional)

For the salad

125g rocket

1 red pepper, sliced

3 tomatoes, sliced

½ small red onion, sliced

1 avocado, peeled, stoned and sliced

1 tbsp extra virgin olive oil

juice of ½ lemon

Heat a large saucepan over a medium heat. Add the olive oil and fry the onion, garlic and chilli for 1–2 minutes, until softened a little. Add the spices and coriander and cook for a further 1–2 minutes. Add the tomatoes, kidney beans and stock. Bring to the boil and cook for 20 minutes over a medium–high heat. You want most of the liquid to evaporate, so keep an eye on it and stir often. Remove from the heat and let it cool a little.

Remove about a third of the kidney beans from the pan and set to one side. Blitz the remaining mixture in a food processor or blender until smooth, then return to the pan, add the whole beans and stir them in. The mixture should be a little stiff. If you let it cool completely, it will be easier to wrap the burritos.

Heat the oven to 200°C/gas 6.

Divide the cheese between the wraps, keeping some back to scatter over the top at the end. Divide the filling between the wraps and roll each one into a sausage shape.

Spread a thin layer of passata over the bottom of an ovenproof dish that's large enough to hold all the burritos snugly in a single layer. Place them inside so they do and drizzle over the rest of the passata. Sprinkle with the remaining cheese and jalepeños, if using. Cover the dish with foil and bake in the oven for 20–25 minutes, remove the foil and bake for a further 5 minutes to brown the cheese.

Toss all the salad ingredients together and serve with the hot burritos.

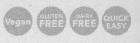

Quick stir-fry with broccoli, seaweed and pak choi

SERVES 4

5g arame
1 tbsp coconut oil
250g pak choi, roughly chopped
1 red onion, thinly sliced
250g broccoli, cut into bite-sized pieces
1 large carrot, cut in half lengthways and sliced at an angle
2cm piece of fresh ginger, finely chopped
1–2 bird's eye chillies, finely chopped
3 garlic cloves, finely chopped
150ml vegetable stock
1 bunch of basil, leaves removed and stalks chopped
1 tbsp tamari (or soy sauce if not avoiding gluten)
100g cashew nuts
250g buckwheat noodles
1 tsp extra virgin olive oil

Prepare the arame according to the instructions on the packet.

Place a wok or a large frying pan over a high heat until it starts to smoke. Add the coconut oil, the vegetables, ginger, chillies and garlic. Keep moving the vegetables around the pan so they don't burn. Cook for 3–5 minutes – lower the heat a little if the vegetables look like they're charring – until cooked but crunchy. Add the stock, basil, tamari and cashew nuts and leave for 30 seconds to warm through.

Meanwhile, cook the noodles according to the instructions on the packet. Refresh in cold water and mix with the olive oil to stop them sticking together.

Serve the stir-fry with the hot noodles.

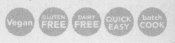

Tofu and squash casserole

SERVES 4

1 tbsp extra virgin olive oil

1 red onion, diced

100g celery, diced

100g carrot, diced

2 garlic cloves, chopped

1 tbsp herbes de Provence

1 litre vegetable stock

2 x 400g tins of white beans, such as cannellini or haricot,
    drained and rinsed

1 tbsp tomato purée

500g butternut squash, cut into bite-sized chunks

100g kale, chopped

350g firm tofu, cut into bite-sized chunks

1 tbsp chopped parsley

Heat a flameproof casserole dish or a saucepan over a
medium heat. Add the olive oil and sweat the onion,
celery, carrot, garlic and dried herbs for 2–3 minutes, until
softened. Add the stock, beans and tomato purée, bring to
the boil, then reduce the heat and simmer for 10 minutes.

Add the squash and cook for a further 10 minutes. Add the kale and cook for 5–7 minutes or until tender. Add the tofu and the parsley, bring to the boil and serve immediately.

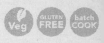

Easy chickpea curry

SERVES 4

1 tbsp coconut oil

1 red onion, sliced

3 garlic cloves, finely chopped

2cm piece of fresh ginger, finely chopped

1–2 birds eye chillies, chopped

1 tbsp mild curry powder

1 tbsp ground cumin

2 tbsp ground turmeric

3 vine tomatoes

500ml vegetable stock

80g kale, chopped

2 x 400g tins of chickpeas, drained and rinsed

2 tbsp chopped coriander

150ml natural yoghurt

300g buckwheat

Heat a large saucepan over a medium heat. Add the coconut oil and fry the onion, garlic, ginger and chillies for for 2–3 minutes. Add the curry powder, cumin and half the turmeric and continue to cook over a low–medium heat for 1–2 minutes.

Cut each tomato into 8 wedges, making sure to keep as much of their juice as possible. Add them to the pan and cook for 1–2 minutes on a medium heat.

Add the stock, kale and chickpeas, bring to the boil and cook for 7–8 minutes over a medium heat.

While the curry is cooking, cook your buckwheat as directed on the packet, with the remaining tablespoon of turmeric stirred into the cooking water.

When the kale is tender, add the coriander and yoghurt to the curry, bring to the boil, then remove from the heat. You might like to add a little more water to loosen the sauce. Serve with the buckwheat.

Lentil and kale moussaka

You can make this up to the point when the moussaka is ready to go into the oven, then leave it in the fridge until you are ready to bake it.

SERVES 4

2 tbsp extra virgin olive oil
1 red onion, diced
2–3 garlic cloves, chopped
100g celery, diced
100g carrot, diced
1 tbsp oregano
1 tbsp rosemary
2 bay leaves
150ml red wine
300ml vegetable stock
1 x 400g tin of green lentils, drained and rinsed
2 x 400g tins of chopped tomatoes
150g kale, chopped
4 large aubergines

For the sauce

60g butter or coconut oil
65g buckwheat flour or plain flour
750ml milk or dairy-free alternative
100g Cheddar or similar hard cheese, grated

In a large heavy-based saucepan, heat 1 tablespoon of the olive oil and cook the onion, garlic, celery and carrot over a medium heat for 2–3 minutes until softened. Add the herbs, wine and stock and bring to the boil.

Add the lentils and tomatoes and bring to the boil, then reduce the heat and simmer for 30 minutes, covered with a lid. Add the kale and cook for a further 10 minutes.

Meanwhile, heat the oven to 200°C/gas 6. Slice the aubergines lengthways into 1cm-thick slices. Brush the slices with the remaining tablespoon of olive oil and place in the oven on a non-stick tray or one lined with greaseproof paper. Bake for 7–8 minutes on each side, then transfer to a plate and set aside. Increase the temperature to 220°C/gas 7.

To make the sauce, bring the milk to the boil in a small saucepan, taking care that it doesn't spill over. Next melt the butter in a separate pan and add the flour. Mix together until you have a mixture that is neither too wet nor too dry. You may have to add a little more flour or butter to achieve this. On a low heat gently cook this for 30 seconds to 1 minute until it leaves the side of the pan. Gradually add the hot milk, stirring continuously until you have a nice thick sauce. Add all but a handful of the cheese, remove from the heat and set aside.

To assemble the moussaka, place a small amount of the sauce in the bottom of an ovenproof dish and spread it around evenly. Cover with a layer of aubergine, then the lentil filling, another layer of aubergine, one more of the filling and a final layer of aubergine. Top with the sauce and sprinkle over the reserved grated cheese.

Place in the hot oven and bake for 15–20 minutes (extend the cooking time by 10–15 minutes if you are reheating from cold). It will be ready when the cheese is nice and browned on top.

JUICES, SMOOTHIES AND OTHER DRINKS

Important note: The juices in this section need to be made in a juicer, and the smoothies in a high-powered blender or smoothie maker.

Pak choi and rocket green juice

This is the first of two alternatives to the classic Sirtfood green juice for when you want to mix things up without losing your morning hit of Sirtfood goodness.

SERVES 1

1 medium (100g) pak choi
a large handful (30g) rocket
a medium handful (15g) watercress
a very small handful (5g) chives
2–3 large green celery sticks (150g), including leaves
1–2 cm piece of fresh ginger
juice of ½ lemon
½ level tsp matcha

Mix the pak choi, rocket, watercress and chives together, then juice them.

Now juice the celery and ginger.

You can peel the lemon and put it through the juicer as well, but we find it much easier simply to squeeze the juice by hand. By this stage, you should have around 250ml of juice in total, perhaps slightly more.

It is only when the juice is made and ready to serve that you add the matcha. Pour a small amount of the juice into a glass, then add the matcha and stir vigorously with a fork or teaspoon. Once the matcha has dissolved, add the remainder of the juice. Give it a final stir and your juice is ready to drink.

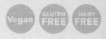

Watercress and lime green juice

Another alternative to the classic Sirtfood green juice to add variety to your morning green juice repertoire.

SERVES 1

3 large handfuls (75g) watercress
2–3 large green celery sticks (150g), including leaves
1 green apple
1–2 cm piece of fresh ginger
juice of 1 lime
½ level tsp matcha

Juice the watercress first, then juice the celery, apple and ginger.

You can peel the lime and put it through the juicer as well, but we find it much easier simply to squeeze the juice by hand. By this stage, you should have around 250ml of juice in total, perhaps slightly more.

It is only when the juice is made and ready to serve that you add the matcha. Pour a small amount of the juice into a glass, then add the matcha and stir vigorously with a fork or teaspoon. Once the matcha has dissolved, add the remainder of the juice. Give it a final stir and your juice is ready to drink.

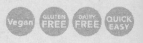

Carrot apple and ginger smoothie

You can swap the water either for coconut water or unsweetened almond milk for a slightly different taste.

200ml water
25g carrot, grated
90g unpeeled apple, sliced
5g fresh ginger, sliced
10g walnuts
1 pitted Medjool dates
½–1 tsp ground turmeric, according to taste

Place all the ingredients in a high-powered blender and blitz until smooth.

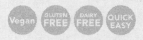

Berry and banana smoothie

You can swap the water either for coconut water or unsweetened almond milk for a slightly different taste.

150ml water
70g strawberries, hulled and halved
40g raspberries
40g blackberries
50g banana, sliced
10g walnuts

Place all the ingredients in a high-powered blender and blitz until smooth.

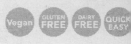

Green tea and rocket smoothie

You can swap the water either for coconut water or unsweetened almond milk for a slightly different taste.

200ml water
50g banana, sliced
25g pitted Medjool dates
15g rocket
1 tsp matcha
5g parsley

Place all the ingredients in a high-powered blender and blitz until smooth.

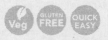

Chocolate strawberry milk

This can be made vegan and dairy free if you use a non-dairy milk such as almond or soya.

150g strawberries, hulled and halved
1 tbsp cocoa powder (100 per cent cocoa)
10g pitted Medjool dates
10g walnuts
200ml milk or dairy-free alternative

Place all the ingredients in a blender and blitz until smooth

Pineapple lassi

200g pineapple, cut into chunks
150g Greek yoghurt
4–5 ice cubes
1 tsp ground turmeric

Place all the ingredients in a high-powered blender and blitz until smooth. If the mixture is too thick, simply add a little water and blend until you have your desired consistency.

Strawberry lassi

150g strawberries, hulled and halved
150g Greek yoghurt
4–5 ice cubes
pinch of ground cardamom

Place all the ingredients in a high-powered blender and blitz until smooth. If the mixture is too thick, simply add a little water and blend until you have your desired consistency.

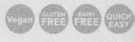

Sirt Shot

This is not a drink for the faint of heart. It packs an invigorating punch and has some serious heat. It's a perfect switch when you're looking for something very different from your normal green juice, or just want to give yourself a kick-start. Bottoms up!

3–5cm (10g) turmeric root, peeled
4–6 cm (25g) fresh ginger, peeled
½ medium (70g) apple, unpeeled
juice of ¼ lemon
pinch of black pepper

Juice the turmeric, ginger and apple.

You can peel the lemon and put it through the juicer as well, but we find it much easier simply to squeeze in the juice by hand.

Grind in a dash of black pepper and stir your juice.

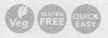

Chilli hot chocolate

This can be made vegan and dairy-free if you use a non-dairy milk such as unsweetened almond or soya.

SERVES 1

1 bird's eye chilli
250ml milk or dairy-free alternative
1 tsp cocoa powder (100 per cent)
35g dark chocolate (70 per cent cocoa solids), grated
1 tsp date syrup

Cut the chilli in half and chop it into 6 or 7 pieces.

Place in a small saucepan along with the remaining ingredients and bring to a gentle boil over a medium–high heat, stirring occasionally so as not to let the milk burn or boil over.

Simmer gently for 2–3 minutes, then remove from the heat and leave to infuse for 1 minute. Strain through a fine sieve and serve.

Hot turmeric milk

We strongly recommend using full-fat milk for this recipe as the fat content increases the absorption of the active nutrients in turmeric. The heat and black pepper support this.

SERVES 1

275ml full-fat milk
1 tsp ground turmeric
1cm piece of fresh ginger, chopped or grated
1 tbsp date syrup
pinch of black pepper

Place the milk, turmeric and ginger in a saucepan and bring to a gentle boil over a medium–high heat, stirring occasionally and taking care not to let the milk burn or boil over.

Reduce the heat to a simmer and cook very gently for a further 5 minutes; this will reduce the bitterness of the turmeric. Add the date syrup and black pepper, then remove from the heat. Leave to infuse for a further 5 minutes, covered with a lid, then strain through a fine sieve and serve.

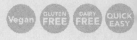

Vegan mocha milk

SERVES 1

250ml dairy-free milk

50g vegan dark chocolate (at least 70 per cent cocoa solids), grated

1 tsp instant coffee granules (or more depending on how strong you want it)

1 tsp date syrup

Place all the ingredients in a saucepan and bring to a gentle boil over a medium–high heat, stirring occasionally and taking care not to let the milk burn or boil over. Reduce to a simmer and serve once all the chocolate has melted.

DESSERTS

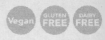

Vanilla and lemon vegan cheesecake

You can make one large cheesecake in a 20cm spring-form cake tin or individual ones in silicon muffin moulds. In the latter case, the number made depends on how large you make them.

SERVES 8–12

200g cashew nuts
160ml almond, coconut or soya milk
100g coconut oil
100g pitted Medjool dates
1 lemon
seeds from 1 vanilla pod

For the base

100g walnuts
75g pitted Medjool dates, roughly chopped
15g buckwheat flakes

Optional toppings

150g strawberries, chopped
150g blueberries
150g vegan dark chocolate (70 per cent cocoa solids), grated

Soak the cashews in the milk and set aside while you prepare the base.

For the base, place the walnuts in a food processor and blend to a fine powder. Add the dates and buckwheat and blend until you have a crumb-like texture.

Line the bottom of your chosen tin mould with the crumb mixture and press it down firmly to form a solid layer. Place in the fridge.

Tip the cashews and their soaking milk, the coconut oil and dates into a blender and blitz for 2–3 minutes, until you have a smooth paste. Using the finest grater you have, grate the zest of the lemon, then juice the flesh. Stir both into the paste along with the vanilla seeds.

Pour the paste over the chilled base(s) and smooth the top with the back of a spoon. Place in the freezer for 2–3 hours, until set; the time depends on the size of your mould. They are a little hard if you serve them straight from the freezer, so take them out at least 30 minutes before serving.

If you are using silicone muffin moulds simply pop them out of the moulds. If you are using a tin, run a sharp knife around the edge then release the spring. Add one of the toppings if you wish, or enjoy the cheesecake on its own.

Date and mocha cups

SERVES 6

375ml milk or dairy-free alternative
500g pitted Medjool dates, chopped
seeds from 1 vanilla pod or 1 tsp vanilla extract
½ tbsp strong instant or espresso coffee granules
2 medium egg yolks
1 tbsp cornflour
100g dark chocolate (70 per cent cocoa solids)

TO SERVE (OPTIONAL)

½ tbsp cocoa powder (100 per cent)
walnut halves, chopped

Have ready six 7.5cm ramekins.

Pour 325ml of the milk into a heavy-based saucepan.
Add the dates and heat gently, stirring from time to time
to avoid it sticking to the bottom of the pan. Stir in the
vanilla and coffee until the granules have dissolved.

Meanwhile, combine the egg yolks, cornflour and remaining 50ml of milk in a bowl. Place the chocolate in a heatproof bowl set over a pan of simmering water, making sure the base of the bowl doesn't touch the water, and leave it to melt. As soon as it has melted, remove it from the heat.

As the milk is coming to the boil, immediately remove it from the heat and whisk in the cornflour mixture. The milk should start to thicken straight away. Return the pan to a very low heat and cook for a further couple of minutes until you have a custard-like consistency.

Pour the custard over the melted chocolate and whisk until you have a nice glossy finish. Pour into the ramekins and allow to cool before placing in the fridge. Chill for at least 2 hours.

Serve the cups as they are, or you could dust with the cocoa powder or sprinkle over the toasted walnuts.

Chocolate popcorn cakes

These cakes couldn't be easier to make but should be eaten on the day they are made or they go a little soft. If you want to make them vegan and dairy-free use a non-dairy milk and ensure the brand of chocolate you use contains no milk solids.

MAKES 8

70g popping corn
1 tbsp coconut oil
150g dark chocolate (70 per cent cocoa solids)
115ml milk or dairy-free alternative
55g pitted Medjool dates, finely chopped
35g walnuts, finely chopped

Place a heavy-based saucepan with a tight-fitting lid over a medium heat. Mix the corn and oil together, then add the mixture to the hot pan and cover with the lid. Shake the pan to keep the corn moving inside it. As soon as it starts to pop, turn up the heat and keep shaking the pan as much as you can with the lid still on. Once the popping calms down to around 2–3 seconds between each pop, remove the pan from the heat and empty it into a bowl. Discard any unpopped kernels, leave to cool.

Place the chocolate in a heatproof bowl set over a pan of simmering water, making sure the base of the bowl doesn't touch the water, and leave it to melt. As soon as it has melted, remove it from the heat and whisk in the milk, little by little, until you have a nice glossy ganache. Stir the dates and walnuts into the chocolate, mixing thoroughly or the dates will clump together.

When the popcorn has cooled, mix it through the chocolate with a spatula, taking care not to overwork it. Spoon into cupcake cases and refrigerate for 1½–2 hours before serving.

Sirt sticky date pudding with toffee sauce

This can be made vegan and dairy-free if you use the coconut oil option instead of butter. If you can't buy ground walnuts, simply place the required weight of nuts in a food processor and blitz until you have a sandy texture.

SERVES 4–6

250g pitted Medjool dates
2 tsp bicarbonate of soda
200g ground walnuts
50g buckwheat flour, sifted
100g unsalted butter or coconut oil, plus a little extra for greasing

For the toffee sauce

200ml coconut cream
100g pitted Medjool dates
150ml water
75g unsalted butter or coconut oil

Heat the oven to 170°C/gas 3½. Lightly grease a 20cm square baking tin.

For the pudding, pour 200ml of boiling water over the dates and leave them to soak for 5–10 minutes.

Once soaked, place the dates and their soaking liquid in a food processor and pulse 7–8 times or until you have a rough paste. Add the bicarbonate of soda and pulse again.

Add the ground walnuts, flour and butter. Blitz until you have a nice smooth paste.

Scoop the mixture into the prepared tin and smooth the top, then transfer to the oven and bake for 30 minutes. (If you prick the middle with a wooden skewer it should come out clean.)

While the cake is baking make your sauce. Place all the ingredients in a small saucepan and bring to the boil. Remove from the heat and set aside for 5–10 minutes to cool a little, then blend, to a smooth sauce. Depending on the brand of coconut cream used, you might have to add a little water if it comes out too thick.

Once the pudding is ready, return the sauce to the saucepan to warm through and serve poured over the warm pudding.

Buckwheat chocolate chip cookies

MAKES ABOUT 20

120g dark chocolate (70 per cent cocoa solids), plus an
    extra 75g broken into chips (cacao nibs can be used
    instead)
20g cocoa powder (100 per cent)
125g buckwheat flour
1 tsp bicarbonate of soda
100g unsalted butter, at room temperature
2 medium eggs
2 tbsp date syrup
1 tsp vanilla extract
125g pitted Medjool dates, finely chopped

Place the 120g of chocolate in a heatproof bowl set over
a pan of simmering water, making sure the base of the
bowl doesn't touch the water, and leave it to melt. Once
melted, remove from the heat and set aside.

Sift the cocoa powder and flour into a bowl, then add
the bicarbonate of soda.

Using a stand mixer fitted with the K attachment or your fingers, blend or rub the butter into the flour mix. When you have an even consistency, add the eggs, syrup and vanilla extract and mix well. Stir in the melted chocolate, dates and chocolate chips.

Lay a 50–60cm sheet of cling film on your work surface. Place the chocolate mixture in the middle and spread it out so it is oblong in shape. Using the cling film to help you, roll the mixture into a sausage shape about 4–5cm in diameter. As you are rolling, twist the ends of the film to make a tight shape. Once you have a tight cylinder, chill the dough for 1 hour. Alternatively, you could just spoon the mixture directly on to a greaseproof-lined baking tray in 4–5cm rounds if you find this easier.

Heat the oven to 170°C/gas 3½. Once chilled, cut the rolled dough into 1cm-thick discs and place on a tray lined with greaseproof paper.

Bake the cookies for 8 minutes. Leave to cool on the tray for 5 minutes, then transfer to a wire rack to cool completely. Any mixture you do not use can be kept in the freezer for up to 3 months as long as it is properly wrapped in cling film.

Quick strawberry mousse

The key to this dessert is to use really ripe, delicious fruit. If you are looking for a more solid consistency, keep it in the fridge for a few hours before serving.

SERVES 4

500g strawberries, hulled
200g (2 medium) bananas
100g Greek yoghurt
cacao nibs, to finish (optional)

Place all the ingredients except the cacao nibs in a blender and blitz until smooth. Transfer to bowls or ramekins and serve immediately, or refrigerate until needed.

Sprinkle over some cacao nibs to serve, if you wish.

Chocolate-dipped strawberries

SERVES 4

70g dark chocolate (85 per cent cocoa solids)
½ tsp vanilla extract
20 strawberries

Place the chocolate in a heatproof bowl set over a pan of simmering water, making sure the base of the bowl doesn't touch the water, and leave it to melt. Add the vanilla extract and stir gently, then remove from the heat.

Line a baking tray with greaseproof paper. Dip the strawberries in the melted chocolate, then put them on the paper and refrigerate for 1 hour before serving.

Hot chocolate pots

MAKES 4–6

5g butter or coconut oil, for greasing
100g dark chocolate (70 per cent cocoa solids)
50ml date syrup
125g butter or coconut oil
4 medium eggs, separated
50g cocoa powder (100 per cent)
pinch of sea salt
1 tbsp cacao nibs

Heat your oven to 180°C/gas 4. Lightly grease four or six 6cm ramekins (depending on how deep you want your puddings).

Place the chocolate, syrup and butter in a heatproof bowl set over a pan of simmering water, making sure the base of the bowl doesn't touch the water, and leave to melt. Once combined, remove from the heat and set aside to cool.

In a stand mixer or using a hand whisk, whisk the egg yolks on a high speed until they double in size and turn a creamy colour. Sift over the cocoa powder and salt and mix at a lower speed until they are thoroughly combined.

In a separate bowl, whisk the egg whites at a high speed until they form soft peaks – you don't want them solid.

Gently fold the yolk mixture into the chocolate. Fold in about one third of the egg whites to loosen the chocolate mixture, then very gently fold in the remainder. You want to keep the air bubbles in the egg white as these are what will make the mixture rise.

Spoon the mixture into the ramekins, or use a piping bag. Gently transfer the mix into the bag and pipe it into the ramekins, leaving a 1cm gap at the top. Use the back of a spoon to level them off, then sprinkle with the cacao nibs.

Bake for 10–12 minutes. They should be nicely risen and cooked on the outside but molten in the middle. Serve immediately but be careful as they will be very hot!

Glossary

Antioxidant (dietary) A substance, either man-made or found naturally in food, which when consumed reduces the physical stress on the cells in our bodies.

Autophagy The process by which our cells break down and recycle waste material and debris in order to use it for fuel. Autophagy is increased during periods of cellular stress (see page 22).

Blue Zones Select geographical regions of the world where people eat diets rich in Sirtfoods and live extraordinarily long, healthy and happy lives.

Caloric restriction A dietary regime where people purposely reduce their food intake in an attempt to lose weight, improve health and extend lifespan.

Circadian rhythm Our natural body clock, which runs on a 24-hour cycle and regulates the activity and efficiency of many important physiological processes, such as sleep and how we process food, according to the time of the day.

DHA (Docosahexaenoic acid) One of two crucial omega-3 fatty acids (alongside EPA), found primarily in oily fish and marine plants such as algae, which enhances the activity of our sirtuins and improves overall health.

EPA (Eicosapentaenoic acid) One of two crucial omega-3 fatty acids (alongside DHA), found primarily in oily fish, which enhances the activity of our sirtuins and improves overall health.

Gene Made up of DNA, the blueprint of our body; when activated, a gene signals the body to produce protein, which changes how the cells work.

Hormesis A biological phenomenon whereby exposure to something that is bad for us in high amounts is actually beneficial in small and moderate quantities. Examples include exercise and fasting.

Inflammaging A persistent, low-grade inflammation that occurs with ageing and increases our risk of many chronic diseases.

Intermittent fasting An umbrella term for any diet that is characterised by alternating periods of caloric restriction (fasting days) and ad lib feeding. Fasting days are usually limited to between 1 and 3 days a week, so this practice is usually more intense than normal caloric restriction.

Leucine An essential amino acid found in dietary protein. It has a potent effect in enhancing the benefits of Sirtfoods, so a Sirtfood diet should also be protein-rich.

Master Regulator A gene, or something that influences a gene, at the top of a hierarchy that regulates and controls other genes below it.

Metabolism All of the biochemical reactions taking place within a cell that help maintain life.

Mitochondria Tiny structures within a cell that break down nutrients and generate energy. They power the cell to carry out its functions. Muscle cells require a lot of energy, so are particularly rich in mitochondria.

mTOR (mammalian target of rapamycin) A vital growth promotor in the body, but its activity needs to be kept in check or else disease can occur. Its activity is highly influenced by the food we eat.

Muscle Gain Adjusted Weight Loss A method for calculating weight loss where reported weight loss results are not penalised if there has been a desirable increase in muscle. This is a much more accurate way of reflecting changes to overall body composition than simply weight loss alone.

PGC1 alpha (Peroxisome proliferator-activated receptor-gamma coactivator 1 alpha) A key regulator of energy metabolism that stimulates the creation of mitochondria (see above) in our cells.

Polyphenols A vast group of natural chemicals found in plants, which are part of a plant's defences against environmental stresses. When consumed, certain polyphenols switch on our sirtuin genes and give rise to the many benefits of the Sirtfood Diet.

PPAR-γ (peroxisome proliferator-activated receptor-γ) A key regulator of metabolism in our cells that switches on genes involved in synthesising and storing fat.

Sirt-1 The most thoroughly researched of the sirtuin family of genes, and the most important for targeting weight loss. It is activated when cells are stressed, and has numerous health and anti-ageing effects.

Sirtfood A food particularly rich in specific polyphenols that, when we consume them, are able to activate our sirtuin genes.

Sirtuin An ancient family of genes that exist in all of us and are activated when our cells are put under stress. Sirtuins play an important role in health, disease prevention and ageing. In humans, there are seven different sirtuins (Sirt-1 to Sirt-7). Of these Sirt-1 and Sirt-3 are the two most important sirtuins involved in energy balance.

Stem cell A special type of cell that can grow into any type of cell found in the body.

Western diet The typical diet representative of industrialised, modern eating patterns, and the antithesis of that found in the Blue Zones (see page 265). A Western diet is characterised by a high consumption of processed and refined foods and a notable lack of nutrient-rich plants, especially Sirtfoods.

Xenohormesis The biological phenomenon whereby humans can piggyback on the stress responses of plants and experience a wealth of benefits by consuming the polyphenols they produce.

Index

Acknowledgements

We'd like to extend a heartfelt thank you to all of our willing recipe testers, for their culinary endeavours, trusty taste buds and invaluable feedback. And thank you to KX Gym, who continue to lead the way in nutritional excellence in the UK and show that healthy food and great taste go hand in hand.

Aidan would like to say a massive thanks to Carmel, Catherine, Colin, Elaine, Karen and Linda, as well as a special thanks to Emily, James and Rachel who ensured that children's taste buds were especially well catered.

Glen would like to say a huge thank you to Louise, Betty, Adam, Matt and Ruth, along with Rachel and all her recipe-testing friends; not forgetting the ever enthusiastic yet brutally honest child tasting duo, Olly and Obie.

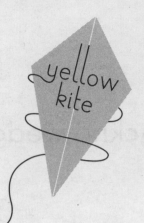

yellow
kite

books to help you live a good life

Join the conversation and tell
us how you live a #goodlife

🐦 @yellowkitebooks
f YellowKiteBooks
📌 Yellow Kite Books
📷 YellowKiteBooks